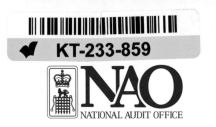

NAO
NATIONAL AUDIT OFFICE

The Challenge of Hospital Acquired Infection

Karen Taylor, Rosalind Plowman and Jennifer A Roberts

About the Authors

Karen Taylor is an Audit Manager on the Health VFM Area of the National Audit Office. She has a BSc Honours degree in Biological Sciences and is a member of the Chartered Institute of Public Finance and Accountancy. Karen has specialised in value for money audit since 1986 and is currently responsible for delivering one of the 5 or 6 major value for money investigations carried out each year in the Health Area. Her report and conference on hospital acquired infection had a significant impact, in terms of parliamentary, public, media and departmental interest and in May 2001, Karen was awarded the Public Finance, Public Servant of the Year Central Government award for this work. In the last 12 months, Karen has also produced a VFM report on Educating and Training the Future Health Professional Workforce and is currently undertaking a VFM study of the Management of Health and Safety Risks in NHS Trusts.

Rosalind Plowman is a lecturer in health economics and a member of the Collaborative Centre for the Economics of Infectious Disease at the London School of Hygiene and Tropical Medicine. Rosalind originally trained and worked as a nurse and then studied for a BA in Human Sciences at Oxford University and an MSc in Health Planning and Financing at the London School of Hygiene and Tropical Medicine and the London School of Economics. In 1993 she was appointed project co-ordinator of a study to assess the economic burden of hospital acquired infections and has been involved in research into the economics of infection and the costs and benefits of selected infection control activities since this time.

Jennifer A Roberts is a Reader in Economics of Public Health and Director of the Collaborative Centre for the Economics of Infectious Disease at the London School of Hygiene and Tropical Medicine. Research work on infectious disease includes studies of E.coli O157, Intestinal Infectious Disease, Hepatitis C and Risk and Infectious Disease in Managed Markets that was funded by the Economic and Social Research Council. She was a grant holder and on the Socio-economic costs of Hospital Acquired Infection study and is presently working on projects concerning MRSA.

Contents

Chapter 3: Strengthening the strategic management of hospital acquired infection

29

Chapter 4: Improving information and understanding 51

Chapter 5: Reducing hospital acquired infection by influencing clinical practice 67

Chapter 6: Maintaining the initiative

Appendices

Foreword

E ach year, hospital acquired infections are estimated to cost the NHS around £1 billion and as many as 5,000 patients may die as a result of acquiring one. As head of the National Audit Office, I present 50 or so major reports to Parliament each year as part of my statutory responsibility to provide an independent insight into the performance of public services. My report on the Management and Control of Hospital Acquired Infection in Acute NHS Trusts in England was one of these reports. Published in February 2000, it made a significant impact in raising the profile of this issue. It also made quite an impression with the media who focused their attention on the key facts and figures on Figure on page 2.

In the report we commended the professionalism and dedication of NHS hospital infection control teams and identified many examples of good practice from which others could learn. The report identified the need to improve the strategic management of hospital acquired infection; the lack of information about the extent, cost and impact of hospital acquired infection; and that there is considerable scope to improve prevention, detection and containment measures. However we also concluded that in many NHS Trusts there may be a growing mismatch between what is expected of infection control teams and the staffing and other resources allocated to them.

Prioritisation of resources for dealing with hospital acquired infection is hindered by the general lack of basic, comparable information about rates of hospital acquired infection. We therefore welcomed the Nosocomial *(hospital acquired)* Infection National Surveillance Scheme and the Department's new Clinical Governance and Controls Assurance initiatives which, among other things, focus attention on ways of improving the management and control of hospital acquired infection. In total we made 29 recommendations to help improve the management and control of hospital acquired infection.

Key facts and figures about hospital acquired infection

The top five ways hospital acquired infections can attack

Blood Infections   After Surgery   Urinary infections   Chest Infections   Skin infections

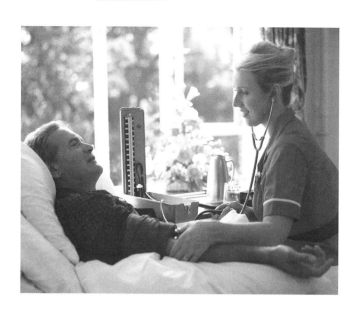

Seven main things about hospital acquired infection

- At any one time 9 per cent of hospital patients have an infection caught in hospital.
- There are at least 300,000 hospital infections a year.
- They are estimated to cost the NHS around £1 billion a year.
- They can mean 11 extra days in hospital.
- The old and young are most likely to catch one.
- Hospital acquired infections may kill: a crude estimate suggests as many as 5,000 patients may die annually as a result of a hospital acquired infection.
- Not all hospital acquired infections are preventable but infection control teams believe that they could be reduced by up to 15 per cent, avoiding costs of some £150 million.

Following publication, Parliament's senior Select Committee, the Committee of Public Accounts, held a public hearing to consider the report. The Committee took evidence from Sir Alan Langlands, the Chief Executive of the NHS at the time, and Professor Liam Donaldson, Chief Medical Officer. In November 2000, the Committee published their findings. The Committee stressed that hospital acquired infections present a serious challenge to the NHS. They recognised that not all hospital infections can be avoided, but emphasised that the NHS needs to do more to establish the extent, cost and effects and to improve prevention. They noted that the Department have launched an array of initiatives to get a better grip on the extent and costs involved, to improve accountability and management in NHS Trusts and to shift the emphasis towards prevention, including monitoring performance and progress. However, the Committee remained unconvinced that the Department have backed up their ambitions with sufficient resources.

The Government's response to the Committee's recommendations drew attention to the numerous initiatives that the NHS has embarked on to tackle the issue of hospital acquired infection. For example, the Department is taking action to improve the data and information available by making surveillance compulsory for all Trusts from April 2001 and is strengthening the performance management system as part of the Clinical Governance and Controls Assurance process. Additional resources have been allocated and other initiatives on antibiotic prescribing, hospital hygiene and education and training have also been launched. The Department accept that the incidence of hospital acquired infection can be reduced significantly with associated cost savings.

In June 2000, I had the pleasure of speaking at a National Audit Office conference that highlighted the conclusions and recommendations from the National Audit Office report and Committee of Public Accounts hearing. A number of excellent speakers from the Department, Public Health Laboratory Service and NHS Trusts explained how they were taking forward initiatives to improve prevention and control of hospital acquired infection. John Denham MP, the then Minister of State for Health, used the opportunity presented by the conference to launch the Government's new UK Antimicrobial Resistance Strategy and Action Plan. Given the wealth of material presented at the conference we agreed to write a book to disseminate this material more widely and also to bring together in one place the numerous Departmental initiatives launched since the publication of my report.

This book should be seen as another step in the National Audit Office value for money audit cycle aimed at promoting better public services. The book highlights the issues that NHS Trusts need to be aware of and the action that they need to take. It looks at the information and resources that infection control teams and clinicians need to have and the actions that everyone who works in a NHS hospital can and should take to help prevent and control hospital acquired infections.

Hospital acquired infection remains a serious issue for health professionals and patients and it is crucially important that the momentum built up so far, is maintained in order to address the serious consequences of hospital acquired infection. This book will be a valuable tool for those tackling an issue of importance to us all.

SIR JOHN BOURN
COMPTROLLER AND AUDITOR GENERAL
NATIONAL AUDIT OFFICE

Chapter 1

Hospital acquired infection: a problem and a priority

Introduction

Hospital acquired infections are infections that are neither present nor incubating when a patient enters hospital but are acquired during a hospital stay. About nine per cent of inpatients have a hospital acquired infection at any one time. Their effects vary from discomfort to prolonged or permanent disability and in a small proportion of cases they may directly or substantially contribute to a patient's death. At the publication of the National Audit Office report, "The Management and Control of Hospital Acquired Infection in Acute NHS Trusts in England",[1] in February 2000, the Comptroller and Auditor General, Sir John Bourn, said:[2]

"Hospital acquired infection can have serious consequences for patients, may be costing the NHS in the region of £1,000 million a year but could be reduced by around 15 per cent across the NHS."

John Denham MP, the then Minister of State for Health, launched the UK Antimicrobial Resistance Strategy and Action Plan[3] at the National Audit Office Conference in June 2000 (Appendix 1) saying that:[4]

"The levels of hospital acquired infection in the NHS are unacceptable. We know there are wide variations in the measures taken by different NHS Trusts to tackle the problem and we believe that some are doing much better than others in tackling the problem."

The Department of Health's (Department's) National Priorities Guidance for 2000/01 - 2002/03[5] identified the control of communicable disease, which includes the control of hospital acquired infection, as one of three "must dos" for the NHS alongside financial control and tackling waiting lists. The guidance refers to strengthening services to prevent and control communicable diseases, especially hospital acquired infection and taking action to reduce microbial resistance.

"The control of hospital acquired infection is a fundamental of hospital care; it is not a priority for this year or the next three years: it's something that should always be there." Dr Pat Troop, Deputy Chief Medical Officer, speaking at the National Audit Office Conference in June 2000.

The NHS Plan Implementation Programme,[6] issued in December 2000, identifies priorities for expansion and reform of the NHS. One of five core requirements is that: "All relevant organisations should ensure that they have effective systems in place, including decontamination, to prevent and control communicable diseases, especially hospital acquired infection so as to minimise the risk of infection to patients and others. Organisations should also take action to control and reduce antimicrobial resistance and meet immunisation targets, including influenza."

Aim of this book

The aim of this book is to help clinical staff and others reduce hospital acquired infection by providing a comprehensive and timely analysis of what is known about the management and control of hospital acquired infection in Acute NHS Trusts. It draws on points made in the National Audit Office report,[1] the Committee of Public Accounts hearing[7] and Departmental response[8] and presentations given at the National Audit Office conference. The book also includes references to recent Department of Health initiatives aimed at improving the management and control of hospital acquired infection.

The National Audit Office value for money examination of hospital acquired infection

The National Audit Office investigation was undertaken in part fulfilment of its responsibility to provide Parliament with independent information, advice and assurance on public expenditure.[1] The issues examined were:

■ whether the overall management and control of hospital acquired infection was being carried out in accordance with existing guidelines and standards;

■ whether infection control arrangements in hospitals were effective and how they could be improved; and

■ what were the factors constraining the application of existing knowledge and realistic infection control measures.

The study methodology and outputs

As neither the NHS nor other interested parties collected comprehensive or comparable data on the management and control of hospital acquired infection the National Audit Office undertook a comprehensive survey of all Acute NHS Trusts (NHS Trusts) between July and December 1998. The National Audit Office also undertook extensive analysis and follow-up work, including visits to a number of NHS Trusts, numerous consultations with stakeholders and extensive literature reviews. Throughout the investigation, an Expert Advisory Group provided advice and guidance to the study team. The National Audit Office report [1], published in February 2000, provided a comprehensive picture of the management and control of hospital acquired infection in NHS Trusts. It also provided details of initiatives that the Department had taken to address hospital acquired infection (Figure 6 in the National Audit Office report is reproduced at Appendix 3).

At the time of the National Audit Office survey, the Department's Regional Directors of Public Health had asked their regional epidemiologists, who provide advice and support to the Department on communicable disease matters, to carry out a survey of the arrangements for the prevention of hospital acquired infection in NHS Trusts. By mutual agreement, and to avoid unnecessary duplication of effort, NHS Trusts were informed in a joint letter from the Department and the National Audit Office that the data collected in the survey would be shared with the regional epidemiologists. In February 2000, based on the analysis conducted by the regional epidemiologists, the Department published an Action Plan (HSC 2000/002) aimed at improving the management and control of hospital acquired infection in NHS Trusts.[9] At the same time the National Audit Office provided a short individual feedback report to each NHS Trust detailing how their performance on several key areas compared with the national and regional picture.

The National Audit Office's overall conclusions and recommendations

The National Audit Office report[1] commended the professionalism and dedication of NHS hospital infection control teams and drew attention to many examples of good practice which were helping to prevent and minimise the problems of hospital acquired infection in individual NHS Trusts. The National Audit Office concluded that:

■ in many NHS Trusts there may be a growing mismatch between what was expected of infection control teams in controlling hospital infection and the staffing and other resources allocated to them;

■ hospital acquired infection was very costly and, to the extent that some of it was preventable, it was possible to improve patient care and save money, but that it would be important for NHS Trusts to justify existing and additional expenditure on infection control against other uses of health resources;

■ evidence based guidelines on the cost effectiveness of measures to reduce hospital acquired infection were lacking and there was scope to improve dissemination of good practice;

■ the prioritisation of resources for dealing with hospital acquired infection was hindered by the general lack of basic, comparable information about rates of hospital acquired infection. The Nosocomial (*hospital acquired*) Infection National Surveillance Scheme[10] and the Department's new Clinical Governance and Controls Assurance initiatives[11,12] which, among other things, focused attention on ways of improving the management and control of hospital acquired infection, were welcome developments; and

■ there were many ways to build upon the work already carried out by infection control teams and others and the Department of Health had recently taken a number of initiatives to raise the profile of hospital acquired infection and improve its prevention and control.

The National Audit Office report[1] detailed 29 recommendations for improving the management and control of hospital acquired infection and urged that these recommendations should be considered quickly, in the interests of better patient outcomes and the release of resources for alternative NHS uses. The recommendations included the following:[1,2]

The Department of Health should:

■ consider revising their 1995 guidance on infection control[13] and ensure that NHS Trusts comply with this guidance and with the controls assurance standards on infection control;

■ consider commissioning research on appropriate staffing levels for the infection control team; and

■ encourage comprehensive participation in the Nosocomial Infection National Surveillance Scheme.[10]

NHS Trusts should:

■ ensure that there is appropriate feedback of surveillance data to clinicians and senior management, who should be encouraged to accept greater ownership for the control of hospital infection; and

■ ensure that infection control considerations are an integral part of bed management policies and that the infection control function is resourced in line with Departmental guidance.

In publishing the report Sir John Bourn said:[2]

"Hospital acquired infections are a huge problem for the NHS. They prolong patients' stays in hospital and, in the worst cases, cause permanent disability and even death. By implementing the National Audit Office recommendations the NHS could make real improvements in the quality of care for patients and could free up significant additional resources for patient care."

The Committee of Public Accounts hearing, their report and the Department's response

The Committee of Public Accounts, the senior Select Committee of the House of Commons questioned the Department on the findings detailed in the National Audit Office report in March 2000. Following the hearing, the Committee produced their report in November 2000.[7] Two overall points emerged from their investigation:

■ The NHS does not have a grip on the extent of hospital acquired infection and the costs involved and is unlikely to have the information needed for a further three to four years. Without robust, up to date, data it is difficult to see how the Department, health authorities and NHS Trusts can target activity and resources to best effect. This lack of data mirrors the Committee's concerns about significant weaknesses in NHS information and systems that have arisen in recent Committee of Public Accounts hearings on medical equipment; inpatient admissions, bed management and patient discharge; and hip replacements. Effective information is essential for good management and effective health care, and central to NHS modernisation.

■ A root and branch shift towards prevention will be needed at all levels of the NHS if hospital acquired infection is to be kept under control. This will require commitment from everyone involved, and a philosophy that prevention is everybody's business, not just the specialists. Leadership and accountability, through the new controls assurance process, are crucial, as is education and training, and monitoring of performance and progress. New investment is also needed. The Department has launched an array of initiatives to help make this happen, but the results have yet to work through, and the Committee was not convinced that the Department had given these initiatives sufficient priority when allocating resources.

In publishing the Committee of Public Accounts report in November 2000, the Chairman of the Committee, David Davis MP, said:[14]

" Hospital acquired infection is both a blight on patients' lives and a major drain on NHS resources. Every year thousands die and £1 billion leaks from NHS coffers. While it will never be entirely preventable there is more the NHS could do. They must now get a grip on this urgently and it is not clear to me that their desire to address the problem is supported by adequate resources."

The Government's response to the Committee of Public Accounts report, published in February 2001,[8] gave details of how the Department are responding to the Committee's nine recommendations. These included the following:

■ surveillance of hospital acquired infection was to be compulsory for all NHS Acute Trusts from 1 April 2001 and that data would be published from 1 April 2002;

- all organisations should have effective systems in place to prevent and control hospital acquired infection[6] and the Department would continue to monitor progress closely to ensure that robust and effective infection control arrangements were in place to protect the health of patients, visitors and staff;

- as part of the controls assurance process, Regional Offices would analyse NHS Trusts self assessments and follow up identified deficiencies;

- an Interdepartmental Steering Group was overseeing and co-ordinating work on the UK Antimicrobial Resistance Strategy following publication of the UK Antimicrobial Resistance Strategy and Action Plan in June 2000;[3]

- new evidence based guidelines for the prevention and control of hospital acquired infection were published in January 2001. These include the standard principles of infection control, including hand hygiene; and

- £31 million was allocated directly to NHS Trusts in July 2000 to secure improvements in the patients' environment, including levels of hygiene and cleanliness, with a further £30 million to be allocated in 2001-2002.

(Appendix 2 provides full details of the Committee's recommendations and the Department's response).

The National Audit Office conference

The findings in the National Audit Office report[1] and Committee of Public Accounts hearing[7] generated significant interest and media attention. In response, the National Audit Office organised a follow-up conference in June 2000 (Appendix 1). The conference provided an opportunity to discuss the main findings of the National Audit Office report and the key themes that emerged during the Committee of Public Accounts hearing. Much of the day was given to presenters with various roles and responsibilities in relation to hospital acquired infection. This allowed delegates to consider many of the Department's existing and planned initiatives and to hear how others were taking forward initiatives at the local level. The conference was attended by infection control nurses and doctors, microbiologists, consultants in communicable disease, regional epidemiologists, consultants in public health medicine and other health care professionals, academics and representatives from the pharmaceutical industry.

The main themes that emerged from the conference were:

■ **The extent and cost of the problem**: There was general consensus that hospital acquired infections are a significant problem for patients and health care systems. They may delay or prevent full recovery and can directly cause or substantially contribute to a patient's death. They are costly to the health sector, patients and their carers. Speakers also noted that a proportion of these infections can be prevented through more effective prevention and control activities, which will lead to improvements in patient outcomes and release resources that can subsequently be used to treat other patients.

■ **Infection control has a low profile in some NHS Trusts and there is a need to strengthen the management framework for hospital acquired infection**: A number of speakers and delegates felt that despite the scale of the problem and the potential for a reduction in rates, prevention and control of hospital acquired infection has generally had a low profile within NHS Trusts. They acknowledged that recent clinical governance and quality assurance initiatives are likely to have a positive impact on the profile and control of hospital acquired infection and that central to this is the role and responsibility assigned to the Chief Executive.

■ **The need for sufficient resources**: Many speakers and delegates considered that the current level of expenditure on infection control was inadequate, and that this, together with pressures from competing objectives, such as reducing waiting lists, was constraining good control practices. While the case for additional resources was made, it was acknowledged that if sustained improvements in infection control are to be achieved there is a need for both existing and new resources to be deployed effectively at local level.

■ **Access to information, including good surveillance data can help improve prevention and control**: Access to accurate data on the incidence of hospital acquired infection varies over time within and between hospitals. Several speakers drew attention to the fact that surveillance of hospital acquired infection is an essential component of an effective infection prevention and control programme but that the methods employed vary. A number of speakers illustrated how surveillance data can be used to identify areas of concern, enabling infection control teams to target these areas as appropriate, and subsequently can be used as a tool to evaluate the outcome of initiatives taken.

- **Infection control is a shared responsibility**: There was general acknowledgement that hospital acquired infection should be the responsibility of all health care workers not just those specifically employed to tackle this problem. However, many health care workers appear to believe that infection control is the responsibility of their infection control team. A number of speakers presented evidence of non-compliance with effective strategies, and poor understanding of the problem suggested that education could assist in raising the profile of hospital acquired infection and improve compliance with infection control activities.

- **Much can be done and is being done to improve prevention and control, including tackling the problem of antibiotic resistance**: Speakers highlighted the fact that prevention and control take many different forms and operate at different levels in the health care system. At the level of clinical practice, hand hygiene is possibly one of the most important interventions. However, there was evidence of non-compliance with this effective, low cost procedure. The global rise of antibiotic resistant micro-organisms was seen as a real threat to effective treatment and there were concerns that some infections are becoming increasingly difficult to treat, and in some rare cases cannot be treated successfully. The need for a concerted effort to tackle this problem through the prudent use of antibiotics, infection control and surveillance was given strong support.

Departmental initiatives launched since the publication of the National Audit Office report

The National Audit Office report drew attention to the fact that, since 1988, the Department have taken a number of initiatives to address hospital acquired infection (the details are reproduced in Appendix 3).[1] As a result the profile given to infection control by the Government and the Department, particularly in the last two years has increased significantly. Since January 2000, when the National Audit Office report was approved for publication, the Department have launched a number of further initiatives which have continued to increase the profile and support improvements in the arrangements for the management and control of hospital acquired infection (**Figure 1**).

Figure 1: In the last 18 months or so there have been a number of initiatives which have helped promote the need for improved management and control of hospital acquired infection

This figure details the key initiatives which have taken place since the National Audit Office report was approved for publication in January 2000. These initiatives have continued to raise the profile of infection prevention and control and ensured that improvements are clearly on the NHS agenda

Feb	2001	The Government's Treasury Minute response to the Committee of Public Accounts report was published.
Jan	2001	Evidence based guidelines commissioned by the Department were published as a supplement to the Journal of Hospital Infection.
Dec	2000	The NHS Plan Implementation Programme was published. One of five core requirements was the need to put in place effective systems to prevent and control hospital acquired infection and reduce microbial resistance.
Nov	2000	The Committee of Public Accounts report on the management and control of hospital acquired infection was published.
Oct	2000	Health Minister, John Denham, announced that all hospitals will be required to monitor levels of hospital acquired infections and that these figures will be published.
July	2000	The Government's NHS Plan included a £31 million campaign to clean up hospitals, based on the introduction of national standards of cleanliness with performance monitored through patient environment action teams.
June	2000	The National Audit Office hosted a Conference on the management and control of hospital acquired infection - 'The Way Ahead'.
		John Denham, Minister of State for Health, launched the Government's new UK antimicrobial resistance strategy at the NAO Conference.
May	2000	The Department adopted and, through NHS Estates, published 'Standards on Environmental Cleanliness' which had been previously issued by The Infection Control Nurses Association and The Association of Domestic Managers.
Mar	2000	The Committee of Public Accounts hearing on the management and control of hospital acquired infection highlighted concerns about the lack of comparable data, poor attention to prevention, impact on the patient and the cost to the NHS.
Feb	2000	The National Audit Office report on the management and control of hospital acquired infection in Acute NHS Trusts in England was published.
		HSC 2000/002 – Departmental guidance on a programme of action to strengthen the management and control of hospital acquired infection was published.
Jan	2000	The London School of Hygiene and Tropical Medicine and Public Health Laboratory Service report on the socio-economic burden of hospital acquired infection was published.

About this book

This book provides an overview of developments in the management and control of hospital acquired infection since publication of the National Audit Office report.[1] It is based on published material, with all sources clearly referenced to the bibliography. The main sources are the National Audit Office report,[1] Committee of Public Accounts report,[7] the Government's Treasury Minute response[8] and relevant Departmental initiatives. The book also uses abstracts from presentations made at the National Audit Office conference to illustrate particular points. The objectives of the book are to:

■ highlight the extent and cost of the problem **(Chapter 2)**;

■ promote improvements in the management arrangements, including examining the adequacy of the resources available for its control **(Chapter 3)**;

■ demonstrate how surveillance can help improve the information base at local and national level **(Chapter 4)**;

■ help improve prevention and control, including tackling the problem of antibiotic resistance **(Chapter 5)**; and

■ maintain the initiative, recognising the actions taken by the Department, and summarising the actions that are needed to ensure that the management and control of hospital acquired infection are improved and lead to reductions in the extent and cost of hospital acquired infection, with associated reductions in mortality and morbidity **(Chapter 6)**.

The authors of this book are:

■ **Karen Taylor**, Audit Manager at the National Audit Office who was responsible for the National Audit Office study design, fieldwork and report[1] and who also put together the programme for the the National Audit Office conference;

■ **Rosalind Plowman**, lecturer in health economics at the London School of Hygiene and Tropical Medicine and an author of the report: The socio-economic burden of hospital acquired infection;[15] and

■ **Jennifer A. Roberts**, Director of the Collaborative Centre for the Economics of Infectious Disease at the London School of Hygiene and Tropical Medicine and an author of the report: The socio-economic burden of hospital acquired infection.[15]

Special thanks to Dr Andrew Pearson, head of the Nosocomial Infection Surveillance Unit at the Public Health Laboratory Service who provided specialist advice and guidance throughout the production of the book. Thanks also to Judith Sedgwick, Senior Nurse in Infection Control at the Public Health Laboratory Service who provided valuable input to the final drafting stages. Finally, thanks also to all of the speakers at the the National Audit Office conference (Appendix 1) who kindly agreed to the use of their conference material and, together with the Department, provided feedback on our use of this material and on the overall contents of the book.

Chapter 2
The national burden of hospital acquired infection

Quantifying the extent of hospital acquired infection and its impact on mortality is difficult as, hitherto, NHS Trusts have not been required to publish data on rates and such data that had been published were limited and not comparable.[1] While most Trusts have undertaken some form of surveillance to detect hospital acquired infection there have been wide variations in the criteria used to define infections, the types of infections monitored, surveillance methods used and the ways infection rates were calculated. Attributing costs to hospital acquired infection is complex and uncertain and getting accurate data on mortality is difficult because in complex cases the causes are multiple.[7]

This chapter details what is known, nationally, about the extent and cost of hospital acquired infection, it covers:

■ the definition and causes of hospital acquired infections;

■ the significance of the problem for the NHS;

- at any one time 9 per cent of in-patients have a hospital acquired infection;

- over 300,000 in-patients a year acquire one or more infections;

- a rough estimate suggests that as many as 5,000 in-patient deaths annually may be directly attributable to hospital acquired infections;

- hospital acquired infections may be costing the NHS as much as £1 billion a year; and

- some infections present post-discharge but few Trusts know the extent of such infections;

■ the fact that while there will always be an irreducible minimum level of hospital acquired infection, there is scope to reduce the incidence of hospital acquired infection and as such reduce the burden on health sector resources; and

■ examples of ways in which hospital infections can affect the Trust's other objectives such as bed management, waiting lists and clinical negligence claims.

The definition and causes of hospital acquired infections

As already noted, hospital acquired infections are infections that are neither present nor incubating when a patient enters hospital but are acquired during a hospital stay. The infection may present while the patient is in hospital or in the community, following discharge from hospital. An infection occurs when a micro-organism (bacterium, a protozoan, a virus or a fungus) invades a susceptible host and causes disease. The majority of hospital acquired infections are caused by bacteria. Some infections are derived from the patient's own normal flora as a result of a change in the relationship between the micro-organism and the patient. Others result from the transfer of micro-organisms from other patients or from the environment. Infective agents may enter the body via the gastro-intestinal tract, genito-urinary tract, respiratory tract, the blood stream or via an open wound. If they are transferred in sufficient numbers and the patient is susceptible to infection, then an infection is likely to occur.[16]

The very old and the very young, who have less efficient immune systems, are particularly susceptible to hospital infections as are patients undergoing therapies that suppress the immune system, such as patients undergoing organ transplantations, patients receiving chemotherapy and patients with diseases affecting the immune systems. Key risk factors include the severity of the underlying illness, the use of invasive procedures, the presence of medical devices and the length of stay in hospital.[1] Some patients in hospital have so many risk factors that a hospital acquired infection cannot always be prevented. However by reducing risks infection rates may be reduced.

A hospital acquired infection may result in pain and anxiety and reduce the health status of the patient concerned. The relationship is complex and the impact will depend on the type of infection (for example, the site and micro-organism involved), its severity and the underlying health status of the individual. For example, a urinary tract infection in a young patient may have little impact but in an elderly patient the effect may be more substantial. A wound infection following a prosthetic hip replacement may have long term consequences for the individual concerned, while in a hernia repair operation the effects of infection may be minimal and short lived.[15]

Antibiotics have been used successfully for more than 50 years to control and treat bacterial infections. However, their use has led to the emergence of strains of bacteria resistant to widely used antibiotics. These drug resistant bacteria are commonest in hospitals where high levels of antibiotic usage allow the drug resistant organisms to evolve and where close concentrations of people with increased susceptibility to infection allow the organisms to spread.[1]

The significance of the problem for the NHS

At any one time 9 per cent of in-patients have a hospital acquired infection

At any one time, an estimated nine per cent of hospitalised patients have an infection that they acquired during their hospital stay. However the prevalence of hospital acquired infection varies considerably with specialty. Urinary tract, lower respiratory tract and surgical wound infections are the three most frequent types of infection observed. (**Figure 2**).[17]

Over 300,000 in-patients acquire one or more infections each year

In evidence to the Committee of Public Accounts hearing the Department acknowledged that hospital acquired infections were a very serious issue but that the information available was limited.[7] The most widely quoted estimate was derived from a study of 19 hospitals (Glynn et al)[18] which looked at adult patients who acquired pneumonia, bacteraemia, and urinary tract infections within four main specialties: general surgical, general medical, gynaecology and orthopaedic; over the period August 1994 to September 1995. By extrapolating their audit findings, the study team estimated that there would have been approximately 60,000 such infections in England and Wales during the year. Because this estimate took no account of cases of hospital acquired infection that might have occurred in specialties not studied and excluded surgical wound and skin infection, which the latest prevalence study suggested accounted for 20 per cent of all hospital acquired infections,[17] the study team estimated that there may be at least 100,000 hospital acquired infections per year.[18] The Department noted that this estimate did not include infections that presented post-discharge and that 100,000 is likely to be an underestimate.[7]

*Urinary tract infections are the most common type of hospital acquired
infection and blood stream infections have the highest associated mortality*

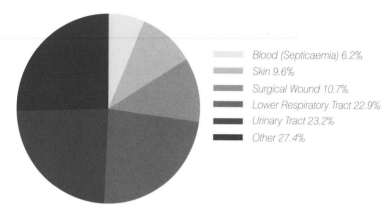

Blood (Septicaemia) 6.2%
Skin 9.6%
Surgical Wound 10.7%
Lower Respiratory Tract 22.9%
Urinary Tract 23.2%
Other 27.4%

Note: 37,111 patients from 157 hospitals were studied over a 15 month period between May 1993
and July 1994 in two month study periods and a mean hospital acquired infection prevalence
rate of 9 per cent (range 2-29 per cent) was calculated.

Source: Second prevalence study Emmerson et al (1996)[17]

A more recent estimate was derived from a study of the socio-economic burden
of hospital acquired infection by the London School of Hygiene and Tropical
Medicine and the Central Public Health Laboratory.[15] The study, which was
commissioned by the Department in 1994, recruited adult, non-day case patients
from eight specialties in one district general hospital and extrapolated the results
to calculate a national estimate. The report, which was published in January
2000, indicated that in 1994-95 at least 321,000 patients acquired one or more
hospital acquired infections which presented during their in-patient phase.

The estimate was limited to adult non-day case patients admitted to the eight
specialties included in the underlying study in NHS hospitals in England:
medicine, surgery, gynaecology urology, orthopaedics, care of the elderly,
obstetrics (limited to patients who had a caesarean section) and ear, nose and
throat. Together they represent 70 per cent of all non-day case admissions per
annum. The estimate did not take into account infections occurring in adult non-

day case patients admitted to the specialties not covered by the study nor did it take into account infections occurring in day case patients, children or neonates or infections which present post-discharge. As such, the 321,000 figure is likely to be an underestimate.[7]

A rough estimate suggests that as many as 5,000 in-patient deaths per year may be directly attributable to the presence of a hospital acquired infection

Hospital acquired infection can result in prolonged or permanent disability and some hospital acquired infections prove fatal.[1] A comprehensive study which took place in the United States of America between 1975 and the early 1980s (Study of the Efficacy of Infection Surveilance and Control Programs in Preventing Nosocomial Infections -Haley et al),[19] estimated that hospital acquired infection was amongst the top ten causes of deaths. There are no equivalent data available in the United Kingdom but, in 1995, a crude comparison by a Department of Health and Public Health Laboratory Service Working Group, estimated that every year some 5,000 in-patient deaths might be as a direct result of acquiring an infection in hospital and, in a further 15,000 cases, hospital acquired infection might be a substantial contributor.[1,13] More recently, the socio-economic burden study suggested that patients with a hospital acquired infection were 7.1 times more likely to die than uninfected patients.[15]

In evidence to the Committee of Public Accounts, the NHS acknowledged that the estimate of 5,000 deaths directly resulting from hospital acquired infections could be on the low side, but the reality was that nobody knows. Getting accurate figures was difficult, because in complex cases the causes of death were multiple. For example, someone undergoing cancer treatment with their immune system suppressed might be susceptible to secondary infection.[7]

Hospital acquired infections may be costing the NHS as much as £1 billion each year

Treating a hospital acquired infection imposes an additional burden on the hospital and may also result in additional costs to general practitioners, district nursing services, and a range of other health care and community services.[1] The socio-economic burden study[15] found that patients with a hospital acquired infection incurred hospital costs that were, on average, three times those incurred by uninfected patients, equivalent to an additional £3,000 per case, and, on average, had a hospital stay that was 2.5 times that of uninfected patients,

chapter two

equivalent to 11 extra days in hospital. Urinary tract infections were the least expensive and multiple infections the most expensive to treat.

The socio-economic burden study[15] used the detailed cost data from the study hospital to derive a national estimate of the cost of hospital acquired infection. This showed that the impact of hospital acquired infection on NHS hospitals is considerable.[1] Hospital acquired infections were estimated to cost the health sector in England as much as £1 billion per annum (**Figure 3**) and utilise 3.64 million bed days, equivalent to an estimated 478,947 finished consultant episodes.[15] While the study included a comprehensive range of costs, extrapolating the results from one hospital across the NHS inevitably has its limitations. Nevertheless, the estimate, which relates to the economic burden associated with the amount of hospital acquired infection occurring in just 70 per cent of all adult non-day case patients, demonstrates that hospital acquired infections use a substantial proportion of scarce resources and remains the only national estimate of costs currently available.[1,7]

Figure 3: The national burden of hospital acquired infection

Hospital acquired infections are estimated to cost the health sector in England as much as £1 billion per annum:

- ■ £931 million relates to additional in-patient hospital care

- ■ £27 million additional out-patient hospital care

- ■ £8 million the cost to general practitioner services

- ■ £21 million the cost to district nurse service

Note: The estimate is limited to the burden of hospital acquired infection occurring in adult, non-day case patients in the following specialties: medicine, surgery, gynaecology, urology, orthopaedics, care of the elderly, obstetrics (caesarean sections only) and ear nose and throat. Patients admitted to these specialities represented approximately 70 per cent of all adult non-day case admissions in 1994/5.

Source; Plowman R, Graves N, Griffin M, Roberts JA, Swan A, Cookson B, Taylor L - The socio-economic burden of hospital acquired infection.[15]

Some infections do not present until after discharge from hospital though few NHS Trusts know the extent of such infections

With moves towards shorter hospital stays, the number of infections that manifest themselves post-discharge is likely to be growing, but few NHS Trusts are aware of their post-discharge infection rates.[1] However, several studies, limited to the incidence of surgical wound infections, suggest that between 50 per cent and 70 per cent of surgical wound infections occur after the patient has been discharged from hospital.[20]

In recognition of the need for effective post-discharge surveillance, the Department funded a Public Health Laboratory Service research study to evaluate post-discharge surveillance methods. Phase 1 was completed in 1997 and Phase 2, which ran from September 1998 to December 1999, was reported to the Department in 2000.[1] The results from this comprehensive study of post-discharge surgical wound surveillance in three NHS Trusts support the findings from previous studies.[1]

The socio-economic burden study team tracked a sample of the patients involved in their study on their release from hospital.[15] The study found that 19.1 per cent of patients who did not present with an infection during the in-patient phase, reported symptoms of, and in some cases received treatment for, an infection manifesting post-discharge that may have been associated with their hospital admission.

In September 2000, the Department established a new NHS Healthcare Associated Infection Surveillance Steering Group to provide them with urgent recommendations on infection surveillance needs at local, regional and national level. This group is also taking forward work on post-discharge surveillance. In January 2001, a UK-wide meeting of consultant microbiologists and others with a key interest in this area was held in Glasgow to review progress and make recommendations.[8]

The extent to which hospital acquired infections can be reduced

Reducing hospital acquired infection would result in improved patient outcomes and the release of considerable resources for alternative use. The National Audit Office estimated that on average 15 per cent of hospital acquired infection could be prevented through improvements in infection control.[1] This estimate was based on a bed-weighted average of responses from 174 infection control teams. The magnitude of resources released inevitably depends upon which infections are prevented and the level of reduction achieved. At the national level a crude estimate by the National Audit Office suggested that a 15 per cent reduction would lead to the release of resources valued at over £150 million.[1,15]

This estimate needs to be treated with some caution as it was derived using the £1 billion estimate extrapolated from the findings in one District General Hospital. However, the Department accepts that the incidence of hospital acquired infection can be reduced significantly with associated costs savings and told the Committee of Public Accounts that it has a wide range of action in hand to achieve this end.[8]

Other NHS Trust healthcare policies can have a significant impact on infection control

Preventing infection can be adversely affected by a Trust's bed management policies

The National Audit Office report emphasised that preventing infection can be adversely affected by other NHS Trust-wide policies, especially bed management practice.[1] The House of Lords Report on Resistance to Antibiotics and other Antimicrobial Agents[21] noted that faster throughput increases risk but is not incompatible with good practice. They explained that this was because faster throughput can itself lead to fewer hospital acquired infections if done in the interests of reducing the overall length of patient stay. However the report went on to note that: "A concomitant of general staff shortages and the pressures created by high bed occupancy is increasing reliance on agency nurses. Agency staff are sometimes poorly versed in infection control and may be unfamiliar with local procedures and, in moving frequently from one place of work to another, they may act as carriers of infection."[21]

A National Audit Office report "Inpatient Admissions and Bed Management in NHS Acute Hospitals", published in February 2000, noted that hospitals with average bed occupancy rates above 85 per cent were at risk of regular bed shortages and periodic bed crises.[22] Furthermore, shorter intervals between the discharge of one patient from a bed and admission of a new patient may increase the risk to patients of hospital acquired infection. Should patients acquire an infection, their extended length of stay may result in bed blocking which would undermine the NHS Trust's attempts at greater throughput.[1,22] At the National Audit Office conference one infection control doctor gave a graphic description of the inter-relationship of infection control and bed management (**Conference abstract 1**).

Conference abstract 1
Infection control should be an integral part of bed management

Problem
Audits throughout the country have shown that hospital beds are contaminated with methicillin resistant *Staphylococcus aureus* (MRSA), vancomycin resistant *Enterococci* (VRE) and a wide variety of other organisms and that they are generally very inadequately cleaned as there is no time to do it properly. There are often situations where the turnover of patients per bed may be as high as three patients in one day. In some situations patients may be taken to the operating theatre on a contaminated bed. One hundred per cent bed occupancy means that you may find a patient about to have a joint replacement next to an emergency admission with discharging pus. Clinical teams may have to visit 15-20 wards during one ward round. Patients may move between several wards on one admission. One hundred per cent bed occupancy therefore compromises the quality of care given to patients. It is associated with poor staff morale and can lead to staff sickness and absence, necessitating bank and agency staff who may have less than optimal skills and limited training in infection control procedures.

Solution
In determining admission policies, NHS Trusts should consider managing elective surgery separately from emergency work. Trusts should monitor indicators such as length of stay in association with hospital acquired infection, staff sickness/absence rates, drug costs and more importantly patient outcomes. The concept should be one of joined up management, with the management of hospital acquired infection seen as a collaborative approach owned by everyone and the need for infection control to be an integral part of bed management.

Source: Presentation at National Audit Office conference by Dr Louise Teare, Consultant Microbiologist at Mid Essex Hospitals NHS Trust

As part of the National Booked Admissions Programme, NHS Trusts are taking forward work on the relationship between demand and supply in order to schedule work more effectively. Central to this is effective bed management and that best practice will be shared through the Modernisation Agency. Although current bed occupancy in general and acute beds is around 83.1 per cent (1999-2000), the NHS Plan provides for an additional 2,100 general and acute beds by 2003-2004 and anticipates that this will reduce the bed occupancy rate to 82 per cent.[8] In July 2001, NHS Estates issued guidance on infection control in the built environment. The aim of this guidance is to help reduce the burden of healthcare associated infection by developing partnerships between architects, designers, builders, healthcare staff and infection control teams both in planning new facilities or renovating older buildings.[23]

Acquiring a hospital infection can result in a clinical negligence claim against the Trust

Hospital acquired infections can result in clinical negligence claims.[1] The Department, however, do not know what costs have arisen from clinical negligence claims from hospital acquired infections.[7] Historically, information on clinical negligence costs has not been collected consistently, and although improvements have been made there are no centrally held data on how many compensation claims the NHS has had where hospital acquired infection was cited as a main or contributory cause. The NHS Litigation Authority is aware that a small but growing number of clinical negligence claims cited hospital acquired infection as a component of the circumstances resulting in a claim being made. The Department told the Committee of Public Accounts that in their view, this appears to reflect the growing incidence of hospital acquired infection in clinical settings generally.

The National Audit Office report "Handling Clinical Negligence Claims in England" (HC 403, Session 2000-2001), published in May 2001, noted that since 1997 the Clinical Negligence Scheme for Trusts in England has had risk management standards for its members.[24] Their purpose is to ensure that risk management is conducted in a focused and effective fashion and makes a positive contribution towards improvement in patient care. The NHS Litigation Authority has revised these standards,[25] drawing on key aspects of the Department's Controls Assurance Infection Control Standards[12] and Health Service Circular 2000/002.[9] The NHS Litigation Authority will begin to assess Trusts against these revised standards during 2001-2002.[8]

Summary

The NHS do not have up-to-date robust information on the extent of hospital acquired infection and the costs involved and are unlikely to have such information for a further 3-4 years.[7] The information that is available indicates that hospital acquired infection is a substantial problem for patients and costs the NHS £100s of millions. Hospital acquired infections also have a significant impact on the other policies within NHS Trusts. The Department have acknowledged the need to improve the information base at Trust level,[7] the subject of Chapter 4 of this book, and accepts that the incidence of hospital acquired infection can be reduced significantly with associated cost savings.[8]

However, as indicated in the Introduction chapter and Appendix 3, the Department have launched a number of initiatives which should ensure that the subject is more firmly in focus, increase its profile and support improvements at the local level. In particular, the NHS Plan Implementation Programme[6] makes it very clear that, as one of the core requirements underpinning the NHS targets set out in the NHS Plan, all relevant organisations must have effective systems in place to prevent and control hospital acquired infection and to control anti-microbial resistance. The rest of this book considers what can be and is being done at the local level and the limitations and constraints to improving the management and control of hospital acquired infection.

chapter two

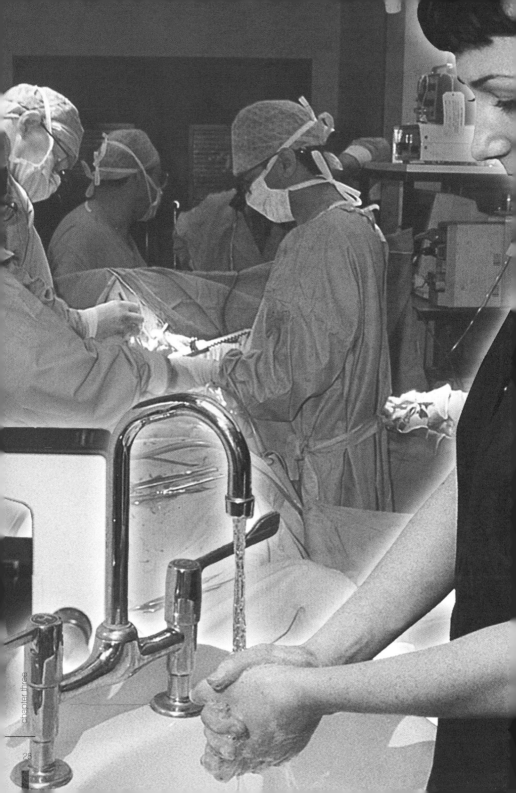

Chapter 3

Strengthening the strategic management of hospital acquired infection

Whilst a number of NHS Trusts have put infection control high on their agenda, the National Audit Office found that health authorities and NHS Trusts generally could do more to improve their strategic management. Also, in many Trusts there may be a growing mismatch between what was expected of infection control teams and the staffing and other resources available to them.[1] This chapter considers the effectiveness of the arrangements for managing hospital acquired infection in NHS Trusts and examines the adequacy of resources available for its control. It highlights the crucial role of the Chief Executive in improving the management and control of hospital acquired infection. The main themes covered are:

■ the complexity of the management framework;

■ the low profile of the management and control of hospital acquired infection in some NHS Trusts;

■ how the implementation of clinical governance, risk management and the controls assurance standards can help improve the management and control of hospital acquired infection;

■ the components of good infection control that need to be in place; and

■ the need for adequate staffing and other resources if infection control is to be more effective.

The NHS Trust management framework for hospital acquired infection is complex

The National Audit Office found that the framework of responsibilities for managing hospital acquired infection is very complex (**Figure 4**).[1] The Department has overall policy responsibility and the Chief Executive of every hospital NHS Trust is responsible for ensuring that effective infection control arrangements are in place and subject to regular review. The key management forum for infection control within NHS Trusts is the Hospital Infection Control Committee, and all acute

Department of Health responsible for:
- Setting overall policy issues in relation to public health matters;
- Managing performance of NHS;
- Issuing policy and implementation guidance;
- 8 regional offices are responsible for surveillance and control of communicable disease and infection in the resident population, including hospitals.

NHS Trust responsible for:
- Ensuring that there are effective arrangements for infection control within the Trust.

Hospital Infection Control Committee responsible for:
- Endorsing all infection control policies, procedures and guidelines;
- Providing advice and support on the implementation of policies;
- Collaborating with the Infection Control Team to develop the annual infection control programme and monitoring its progress

The Hospital Infection Control Committee may comprise:

| The Infection Control Team | Chief Executive or representative | Occupational Health Physician and Occupational Health Nurse | Infectious Disease Physician |

Infection Control Team includes infection control doctor(s) and nurse(s) responsible for:
- Ensuring advice on infection control is available on a 24 hour basis;
- Producing the annual infection control programme in full consultation with the ICC, health professionals and senior managers. This programme will include surveillance of infection and an audit of the implementation and compliance with selected policies;
- Providing education and training on the prevention and control of hospital acquired infection to all grades of hospital staff.

Key

→ Accountability

Source: National Audit Office report[1]

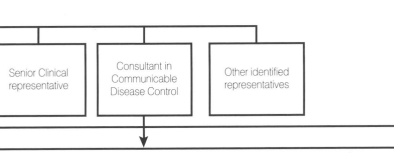

Health Authority responsible for:

- ▦ Ensuring quality of service provided to local population by ensuring adequate infection control arrangements in English hospitals in collaboration with local authorities' environmental health officers;
- ▦ Protecting the public health by controlling communicable disease and infection.

| Senior Clinical representative | Consultant in Communicable Disease Control | Other identified representatives |

nt in Communicable Disease Control responsible for:

lance, prevention and control of communicable diseases and infections in district,
ng management of outbreaks;
ig Health Authorities and Primary Care Groups about service agreements
ction control;
orating with ICT on management of outbreaks both within hospitals and in the community;
ng epidemiological advice.

hospitals should have an infection control team, which has primary responsibility for all aspects of surveillance, prevention and control of infection at NHS Trust level.[1,9]

Health authorities are expected to protect the public health by controlling communicable disease and infection.[13] This responsibility includes ensuring adequate infection control arrangements within hospitals. In addition, since 1988, each health authority has appointed at least one consultant in communicable disease control to maintain a balanced perspective on the wider issues of infection control. consultants in communicable disease control are responsible for the surveillance, prevention and control of communicable diseases and infection within a health authority. They are also:

■   members of a NHS Trust's Hospital Infection Control Committee;

■   required to provide hospitals with epidemiological advice and ensure the wider community perspectives of infection control are understood;

■   expected to collaborate with the infection control team in managing infection outbreaks; and

■   often appointed as "Proper Officer" for the control of infectious diseases within a local authority under the Public Health (Control of Diseases) Act 1984 for which they are accountable to local authorities.

These roles and responsibilities are expected to change under the current NHS reorganisation proposals.

Hospital acquired infection has a low profile in some NHS Trusts

The Department's 1995 guidance[13] stated that communicable disease control and infection should be taken into consideration in every contract which health authorities placed with acute hospitals. Contracts have since been replaced with long term service level agreements. The National Audit Office found that a quarter of service agreements between Trusts and their health authorities did not cover the provision of infection control services.[1,27] Also, where infection control was covered, it was sometimes without input from the people with detailed knowledge about infection control, namely the Trust's infection control team and the health authority's consultant in communicable disease control. The report concluded that lack of detailed specification within service agreements and lack of compliance with them means that many health authorities do not have all the data they need to assess NHS Trusts' performance in improving infection control.[1]

The Department's 1995 guidance required NHS Trust Chief Executives to ensure that, at the local level, effective infection control arrangements were in place and subject to regular review.[13] The National Audit Office found that Chief Executives of most NHS Trusts were not as directly involved as the guidance suggested they should be.[1] In response to questions by the Committee of Public Accounts, the Department acknowledged that in the past many Chief Executives had not been engaged in tackling hospital acquired infection. As a result the issue had a low profile.[7] The Department's new guidance, clearly emphasises that responsibility for ensuring that effective systems are in place is now firmly vested in each Trust and its Chief Executive.[8,9]

At the conference, the National Audit Office commented that, when they commenced their study in 1998, infection control was often referred to as the "Cinderella Service" of the NHS, and that "in some NHS Trusts infection control does not have the profile it merits". The relative lack of involvement of the Trust Chief Executive may provide an explanation for its low status in these NHS hospitals.[1] Speaking at the National Audit Office conference one Chief Executive explained his perspective on this issue (**Conference abstract 2**).

Conference Abstract 2
Improving the management and control of hospital acquired infection requires the full commitment of the Trust Chief Executive

If the problem of hospital acquired infection and its prevention and control is to be given the attention it warrants, the involvement of the Chief Executive is essential. Two main messages that Chief Executives should take account of are:

■ not only should the Chief Executive sit on the Hospital Infection Control Committee, which the National Audit Office report showed was not the case in many Trusts, but they should also have greater visibility at ward level - walking the floor and being seen to be interested in infection control issues; and

■ the need to ensure that the Trust has an adequate budget for infection control, both capital and revenue, and that the Trust Board receives regular feedback on performance.

Source: National Audit Office conference presentation by Graham Elderfield, Chief Executive, Isle of Wight NHS Trust

chapter three

Improving the profile and achieving greater accountability through clinical governance and controls assurance

In February 2000, the Department's Health Service Circular (HSC 2000/002),[9] which was based on an analysis by regional epidemiologists of the results of the National Audit Office survey, detailed action for NHS Trusts to improve the management and control of infection in hospitals. It also built on the clinical governance arrangements and controls assurance standards on infection control, issued in November 1999.[12] The guidance required each Trust to develop an action plan by July 2000 setting out priorities for action and that Trusts should self assess against the controls assurance standards. Together these initiatives are intended to strengthen, considerably, the framework for the management and control of hospital acquired infection including better quality assurance systems and audit.[8]

The clinical governance[11] and controls assurance[12] initiatives are the foundation on which the Department's proposals to strengthen the management structures and increase the profile of hospital acquired infection in NHS Trusts are based. The Minister of State for Health, John Denham MP, speaking at the National Audit Office conference, said that:

> "The clinical governance and controls assurance initiatives should be viewed as one system that ensures quality management within the organisation, that can deliver a service that continuously improves and that is open and accountable. They should be seen as standards set at a national level, standards delivered at local level and standards independently inspected and reviewed."

The clinical governance initiative was launched under HSC 1999/123 'Governance in the new NHS - Action for NHS Trusts and health authorities'.[11] The aim is to provide NHS organisations and health care professionals with a framework which, over the next five years, will develop into a coherent local programme for clinical quality improvement. Its main objective is to ensure that the spirit of clinical governance is embedded within the procedures and systems of accountability within each Trust.

The controls assurance initiative, launched in November 1999,[12] is a process whereby the Trust Boards can assure the public that the Trust operates an effective system of internal control covering key risks. The controls assurance programme complements clinical governance and is intended to ensure the greater involvement of the Chief Executive. Within this programme the aim is that Chief Executive involvement should afford hospital acquired infection and its prevention and control greater visibility. As such this should add weight to efforts directed towards the prevention of infections and assist in the reallocation of resources to what many view as, an under resourced area.[7]

The controls assurance infection controls standard,[12] one of 19 standards issued as part of the controls assurance process, states that: "Acute NHS Trusts should ensure that there is a managed environment which minimises the risk of infection to patients, staff and visitors" (**Figure 5**). The system of controls assurance[11] is intended to ensure that, through a Risk Management Committee, significant risks will be brought to the attention of the Trust Board. Key responsibilities for infection control remain vested in the Trust Hospital Infection Control Committee and an appropriately constituted and functioning infection control team.

Speaking at the National Audit Office conference, Stuart Emslie, Head of Controls Assurance at the Department, commented that:

"Controls assurance is a self assessment process designed to provide evidence that NHS bodies are doing their reasonable best to manage themselves in order to meet their objectives of protecting patients, staff, the public and other stakeholders against risks of all kinds."

The expected benefits from adopting this approach are:

■ a reduction in risk exposure through more effective targeting of resources to address risk areas;

■ improvements in economy, efficiency and effectiveness;

■ demonstrable compliance with applicable laws and regulations;

■ enhanced reputation through public disclosure of achievements in meeting objectives; and

■ better management of risks and, as a result, increased public confidence in the quality of services provided by the NHS.

Figure 5: The Controls Assurance Programme - Infection control criteria[12]

Controls Assurance standard

There is a managed environment, which minimises the risk of infection, to patients, staff and visitors.

Criteria for evaluation

1   Board level responsibility for infection control is clearly defined and there are clear lines of accountability for infection control matters throughout the organisation, leading to the Board.

2   There is an Infection Control Committee that endorses all infection control policies, procedures, and guidance, provides advice and support on the implementation of policies, and monitors the progress of the annual infection control programme.

3   There is an appropriately constituted and functioning infection control team.

4   Prevention and control of infection is considered as part of all service development activity.

5   An organisation wide annual infection control programme with clearly defined objectives is produced by the infection control team.

6   Written policies, procedures and guidance for the prevention and control of infection are implemented and reflect relevant legislation and published professional guidance.

7   There is an annual programme for the audit of infection control policies and procedures.

8   Timely and effective specialist microbiological support is provided for the infection control service.

9   Surveillance of infection is carried out using defined methods in accordance with agreed objectives and priorities, which have been specified in the annual infection control programme.

10 A comprehensive infection control report is produced by the infection control team on an annual basis, reviewed by the Risk Management Committee and presented to the Board.

11 The Infection Control Committee and infection control team have access to up-to-date legislation and guidance relevant to infection control.

12 Education in infection control is provided to all health care staff, including those employed in support services.

13 Key indicators capable of showing improvements in infection control and/or providing early warning of risk are used at all levels of the organisation, including the Board, and the efficacy and usefulness of the indicators is reviewed regularly.

14   The system in place for control of infection is monitored and reviewed by
      management and the board in order to make improvements to the system.

15   The Internal Audit function, in conjunction with the Infection Control Committee and
      infection control team, carries out periodic audits to provide assurances to the Board
      that a system of infection control is in place that conforms to the requirements of this
      standard.

Note: The Controls Assurance standards are subject to regular review. The infection control standard
       is currently being updated and a slightly revised version is expected to be re-issued in
       October 2001. Data source: Infection Control Standards12: Controls Assurance Database -
       www.doh.gov.uk/riskman/htm

Source: Infection Control Standards[12]: Controls Assurance Database - www.doh.gov.uk/riskman/htm

Controls assurance is about "getting the information on the portfolio of risks
(clinical and non-clinical) that exist within an organisation and then using robust
risk ranking and cost benefit methodologies to prioritise the investments that
hospitals need to make to treat the risk". Stuart Emslie recalled a discussion which
he believed helped to illustrate this point (**Conference abstract 3**).

Conference abstract 3
Taking a well calculated risk

An orthopaedic surgeon in an NHS Trust had, as a key objective, the need
to keep to his operating schedules and reduce waiting lists, yet he knew
that there were a number of patients colonised with MRSA and that this
increased the risk of an MRSA outbreak. He weighed up all the risks, the
costs and the benefits and decided, having taken appropriate preventative
steps, to continue to operate. The question the Minister of State for Health
asked Stuart Emslie was whether the surgeon had done the right thing.

His response was that of course he had, as it was a well calculated risk.
To support this view still further he drew attention to the comments of
David Davis MP, Chairman of the Committee of Public Accounts, who has
stated on a number of occasions that he will applaud well thought through
risk taking even when it goes wrong.

*Source: National Audit Office Conference; Presentation by Stuart Emslie, Head of Controls
Assurance Department of Health*

Under the controls assurance standards infection control is a core management responsibility

The controls assurance framework requires that the implementation of controls assurance standards should be monitored at Trust level through internal audit, and nationally by the Commission for Health Improvement and the Audit Commission.[7] In addition, from 2003, statements of assurances are to be presented in the annual reports of NHS Trusts and will be aggregated through regional offices and forwarded to the Department, and the Committee of Public Accounts, so completing the audit cycle.[8]

This requirement for NHS Trusts to assess their performance in relation to infection control against the controls assurance national standards is mandatory, thereby ensuring NHS Trusts give due consideration to this issue. This in turn should help raise the profile of infection and its control.[7] All NHS Trusts were required to complete this baseline assessment by 31 March 2000 and to have developed an action plan by July 2000.[12] The Department's assessment of the first year's results showed that on average NHS Trusts are meeting 53.8 per cent of the infection controls assurance standards (information is held on www.casu.org.uk).

The Chief Executive of each NHS Trust has a duty of care under the controls assurance standards.[7] Every NHS Trust has to live by the standards set by the controls assurance procedure, to report on a regular basis to the Department and to be managed and inspected against the standards. The NHS Plan Implementation Programme[6] has ratified this by making it clear that, as one of the core requirements underpinning the NHS targets set out in the NHS Plan, all relevant organisations must have effective systems in place to prevent and control hospital acquired infection.

Membership of the Trust's Hospital Infection Control Committee needs to be strengthened

To be effective, membership of the NHS Trusts' Hospital Infection Control Committee should include the infection control team, consultant in communicable disease control, occupational health doctor (or nurse) and representatives from various clinical and medical specialties.[13] The Trust Chief Executive or a nominated representative is also expected to be a member of the committee (see Figure 4 on page 30-31).[9,13] The National Audit Office found that while all NHS Trusts had a Hospital Infection Control Committee, membership of the Committee varied as did the attendance of its members.[1] In 1998-99 for example, in 30 per cent of Trusts neither the Chief Executive nor a deputy sat on their Committee. The National Audit

Office concluded that there was a risk that some Hospital Infection Control Committees might not be fulfilling the role envisaged for them and that Chief Executives need to ensure that they were operated as the Department intended and that they or their nominated deputy attended all meetings.[1] Since publication of the National Audit Office report and HSC 2000/002[9] there has been measurable progress in this respect and by January 2001, 91 per cent of Trusts reported that their Chief Executive or Deputy regularly attended Hospital Infection Control Committee meetings.[8]

An effective infection control programme is an essential management tool

The Chief Executives' responsibility for ensuring that there are effective infection control arrangements includes the need to put an effective infection control programme with defined objectives in place.[1,9] The Hospital Infection Control Committee is expected to discuss and endorse this programme and submit it for approval to the Chief Executive.[13] The Committee should also review the progress of the programme, assist in its effective implementation and review the final results. The National Audit Office found that only 79 per cent of Trusts had an infection control programme and of these the Chief Executive approved only 11 per cent.[1]

The Department's February 2000 Action Plan required Chief Executives to work with their infection control teams to ensure that programmes for the control of infection were in place and working effectively by April 2001.[9] In responding to the Committee of Public Accounts report the Department noted that in January 2001, NHS Trusts were actively putting in place infection control programmes for 2001-2002, including measures to address any shortfalls in meeting the Controls Assurance Infection Control Standard.[8]

The key components of an effective infection control regime are detailed in **Figure 6.**[1] These components form part of a jigsaw which the infection control team needs to influence to ensure good infection control practices are implemented and hospital acquired infection rates are reduced (**Figure 7**).

Figure 6: The main components of an effective infection control programme

The main components of an effective infection control programme include:

■ Surveillance of infection - to produce accurate timely information on infection rates and trends, detect outbreaks, inform evaluations of and changes in clinical practice; and assist the targeting of preventative efforts.

■ Provision of education and training - to inform and convince staff of the value of recommended infection control measures.

- Production, review and dissemination of written policies, procedures and guidelines on the NHS Trust's infection control arrangements.

- Monitoring of hospital hygiene - in relation to cleaning, housekeeping, disinfection or sterilisation of instruments and equipment, safe collection and disposal of clinical waste; kitchen hygiene etc.

- Setting and auditing standards of own work, and contributing to the standard setting and audit processes in other clinical and support services to ensure compliance with infection control policies and procedures.

- Contributing to decisions on: the purchase of equipment; plans for alterations and additions to buildings; and the letting of catering domestic and laundry services contracts.

- Specific documented arrangements for dealing with infections, including outbreak control, targeted screening and isolation of patients.

Source: National Audit Office Report[1]

Figure 7: How the components of an infection control programme inter-relate

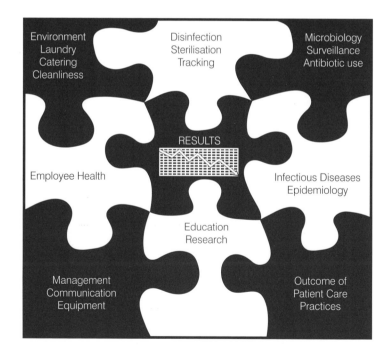

(Diagram by kind permission of Susan Macqueen, Clinical Nurse Specialist Great Ormond Street Hospital for Children NHS Trust)

The availability of adequate resources is key to improving the management and control of hospital acquired infection

There are wide variations in the staffing and other resources available for infection control

Since 1995 there has been a requirement for every NHS Acute Trust Chief Executive to ensure that they have an infection control team comprising an infection control doctor and infection control nurse(s).[13] However interpretation of this requirement has varied in terms of the staffing time dedicated to infection control.[1] The need for all NHS Trust Chief Executives to secure an appropriately constituted and functioning infection control team, including support staffing and resourcing, was included in the Department's programme of action for the NHS (HSC 2000/002).[9]

The National Audit Office report concluded that there may be a growing mismatch between what was expected of infection control teams in controlling hospital infection and the staffing and other resources allocated to them. This conclusion was based on the following findings:[1]

■　There are no Departmental guidelines on infection control staffing. The Royal College of Pathologists[26] suggested that in an average 500 bed District General Hospital the infection control doctor should spend at least half his/her time on infection control (equivalent to one infection control doctor per 1,000 beds). In practice, the ratio of infection control doctors to beds varied widely, with an overall average of one infection control doctor per 2,258 beds. Only 46 per cent of Trusts met the guidelines recommended by the Royal College of Pathologists.

■　In the absence of any guidelines or benchmarks, the one infection control nurse to 250 beds ratio, derived from an American study (Haley et al),[19] was widely quoted by English NHS Trusts in business cases requesting additional staff resources. In practice, however, there was a wide variation in the ratio of infection control nurses to beds (**Figure 8**). The average ratio of infection control nurses' time (in whole time equivalents) to beds in NHS Trusts was one infection control nurse to 535 beds.[1]

Figure 8: The ratio of total number of beds to whole time equivalent infection control nurses in NHS Trusts

The National Audit Office report identified wide variations between NHS Trusts in the ratio of infection control nurses to beds. One American study, in the early 1970s, indicated that there should be one infection control nurse to every 250 beds and this was used as a benchmark in American hospitals. While there is no similar benchmark in England, only 24 out of 218 NHS Trusts met this level, and 11 had over 1,000 beds per nurse.[1]

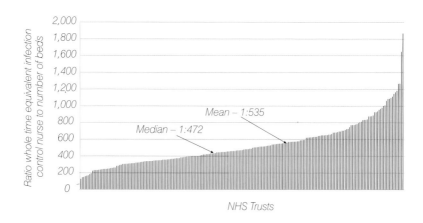

Sample Size: 218 NHS Trusts

Source: National Audit Office Census

■ Over 60 per cent of infection control teams considered that they had inadequate clerical support, with 27 per cent having none. Lack of computer software and hardware was also cited as a major constraint in providing effective infection control. While the Department's NHS Information for Health Strategy, which includes installing electronic patient record systems and reporting results of prescribing, is expected to improve matters, the report noted that infection control teams would need to ensure that they obtain appropriate access.[1]

■ When the Department's 1995 guidance was issued,[13] this stated that the need to comply with the guidelines "should have no financial or manpower implications." Because the resources of many infection control teams, including staff, were allocated for budgetary purposes in other work units it was not possible to draw firm conclusions about relative changes in funding of infection control over time. However, using estimates provided by infection control teams, the National Audit Office noted that after allowing for salary increases, there had been little real terms change in the funding of infection control in hospitals between 1996-97 and 1998-99. During this time, expectations, particularly in relation to a number of resource intensive activities including surveillance, had increased. Also, NHS Trust policies, like movement of patients between beds and between wards, quicker throughput of patients and greater use of invasive techniques had also increased the demand on infection control teams' time and resources.

The Chief Medical Officer, Professor Liam Donaldson, in response to questions by the Committee of Public Accounts, accepted that in staffing infection control teams, a ratio of 1 nurse to 250 beds was a reasonable basis for Trusts to measure themselves against, to look at their own local position and plan what they need to do.[7] In February 2001, the Department told the Committee that since publication of the National Audit Office report there had been some improvements in the staffing and other resources available to infection control teams, with an increase in IT, clerical and secretarial support.[8]

The Department considers that there are rational answers to some of the variations found in the National Audit Office review. For example, infection control teams in very highly specialised children's hospitals are well staffed whereas those at the other end of the spectrum might be NHS Trusts with little acute service activity. There are also variations in practice. For example some Trusts rely heavily on ward-based nurses with specific responsibilities for infection control (known as link nurses), rather than on dedicated teams. The use of link nurses in these Trusts can be effective in controlling infection.[7] Since the National Audit Office study, there had been a number of additional appointments of infection control nurses and Regional Directors of Public Health are continuing to work with Trusts to ensure that, where necessary, improvements are made.[8]

The Department also believe that it is for NHS Trusts and health authorities to decide on the number, grade and mix of staff they require to provide services to patients. However, they propose to hold discussions with the Infection Control Nurses Association and other professional organisations about the development of an assessment tool for NHS Trusts, to help them reach decisions about staffing levels and skill mix required within the infection control team.[8]

Not all infection control teams have their own budget and access to other Trust funds can prove difficult

Quantifying the level of funding currently tied up in infection control is difficult as infection control takes place at many different levels within the hospital (e.g. management, laboratories, and clinical and support services). The Department's 1995 guidance[13] noted that NHS Trusts need to have flexibility in the use of their resources but acknowledged there were advantages for the planning and implementation of an effective infection control programme if infection control teams have a separate budget for routine infection control work. The National Audit Office found that by the end of 1998, some 40 per cent of infection control teams had a separate budget for control of infection in the hospital. However, the amounts allocated varied greatly (from £500 to £1million) which to a degree reflected the varying range of activities the budget was expected to cover.[1]

The recent risk perception study found that the size of budgets allocated directly to the infection control team, or available from other budgets, directly affected the implementation of good infection control practices.[27] For example: in some laboratories microbiologists found it difficult to fund the cost of tests relating to outbreaks and surveillance of MRSA, theatre budgets were often fully committed and on one occasion a surgeon could not find funds to purchase protective clothing needed to perform surgery on patients with multiple resistant tuberculosis. Pressure on beds caused difficulty in closing wards when outbreaks occurred, and at one hospital cleaners were bringing in their own materials because they lacked adequate supplies to do their work properly.

Cleaning budgets and the inadequacy of cleaning is an ongoing theme that emerges from surveys and case studies and has received much media coverage over the last 12 months or so. Speaking at the conference, Graham Elderfield, Chief Executive of the Isle of Wight NHS Trust mentioned that when he asked his cleaning staff whether there was one thing that would make their job easier and more fulfilling, one responded:

"just give me a hoover that works and I could do a better job."

The adequacy of resources for infection control was raised by a number of speakers at the Conference. The main issues raised revolved around the following themes: lack of investment in infection control teams; lack of resources available for infection control teams to do their work; lack of dedicated budgets for infection control teams; the interdependence of budgets; and the overall level of resources available to the NHS and the competing NHS objectives.

New investment promised

The National Audit Office report concluded that hospital acquired infection is very costly and, to the extent that some of it is preventable, it is possible to improve patient care and release valuable resources for alternative use. However, it will be important for NHS Trusts to justify existing and additional expenditure on infection control against other uses of health resources.[1]

Speaking at the conference, the then Minister of State for Health, John Denham MP, noted that historically one of the reasons that the NHS had not done better at tackling hospital acquired infection was a lack of resources. He stated that:

"as the rates of investment in the NHS grow, the NHS must make sure that the resources are in place or re-directed to support infection control."

He drew particular attention to the fact that a key function of the infection control teams is monitoring rates of hospital acquired infection yet some teams do not have access to decent IT equipment and are still using paper based systems. He suggested that the hundreds of millions of pounds being invested in the Information for Health Strategy should ensure, among other things, that infection control teams are provided with the tools to perform their role effectively and efficiently.

The Department acknowledge that the high priority now being given to combating hospital acquired infection needs to be matched by appropriate local funding.[7] They told the Committee of Public Accounts that funding for the NHS as a whole is set to increase by 6.3 per cent year on year. While they do not determine how much of this should be spent at individual hospitals, they expect Chief Executives to spend what is necessary to achieve the targets they have been set. In addition, the NHS received an extra £2 million in 2000-01 and will receive £3 million in 2001-02, primarily to fund development initiatives.[8]

Targeting resources effectively

Convincing those responsible for allocating resources that investment in infection control is money well spent presents a number of difficulties not least because the benefits lie in the avoidance of a potential infection. The Infection Control Nurses Association, in evidence to the House of Lords Select Committee on Science and Technology, stated that:[21]

"It is difficult to justify the costs incurred for an intervention where the successful outcome measure is an event not occurring."

As already noted, the effects of hospital acquired infection can vary from discomfort for the patient to prolonged or permanent disability or even death which makes this a very serious subject in terms of impact on the patients and costs to the NHS. The best estimate available suggests that hospital acquired infection may be costing the NHS as much as £1 billion and that, while attributing costs to hospital acquired infection is uncertain and complex, the potential gross avoidable cost is around £150 million a year.[1,7] While this estimate does not take into account the cost of achieving such a reduction, it does suggest that the benefits of investing in infection prevention and control are likely to be considerable.[1] In terms of bed days released a 15 per cent reduction is equivalent to the release of 546,084 bed days or 71,853 finished consultant episodes.[15]

A number of Trusts have used a business case approach to demonstrate the benefits of investing more resources in infection control

A business case approach, to demonstrate the benefits of investing in an infection control team, can be an effective way of making a case for more resources. Economic models can be developed which take into account the incidence of particular types of infection, the number of patients at risk, the cost of the intervention, the anticipated level of effectiveness of the intervention given 100 per cent compliance and the cost of alternative strategies that aim to increase compliance. Inevitably these models will be based on a number of assumptions informed by the latest literature and local data. Sensitivity analysis can be conducted to test the robustness of the model to changes in the underlying parameters, and the results used to further inform decision-making.

In the absence of data on the effectiveness of the selected intervention, models can be developed that assess the proportion of infections that would need to be prevented to cover the cost of the intervention, and the feasibility of achieving this assessed.

Sixty infection control teams provided the National Audit Office with examples of business cases that they had made for extra infection control resources: 24 of these were successful, 16 were unsuccessful and the decision was unknown or pending in a further 20 cases.[1] Speaking at the conference, the National Audit Office noted that it was impossible to identify what made a successful business case as the allocation of resources inevitably took into account the Trust's other competing priorities. However, the more robust the case the higher the likelihood of success. At the conference, Professor Gary French, Chairman of the Hospital Infection Society and infection control doctor at Guy's and St Thomas' NHS Hospital Trust, demonstrated how he made a business case for additional infection control nurses (**Conference abstract 4**).

Conference abstract 4
A business case for additional infection control resources

The information presented in the business case seeking additional resources included:

- At any one time, about 10 per cent of all patients have a hospital acquired infection[17]. These infections can delay discharge and impose additional costs on the health sector. Estimates suggest that on average hospital acquired infections prolong a patient's hospital stay by 11 days and cost the health sector, on average, an additional £3000 per case.[15]

- A crude estimate suggests that hospital acquired infections cause around 5,000 in-patient deaths per annum and are a substantial contributing factor in a further 15,000 deaths. If so, they kill more people every year than road accidents or suicides.[13]

- It is similar to cancer in that the public is frightened of it as it can kill and yet it is partially preventable.

- It affects waiting lists, delays operations and blocks beds.

- It can contribute to the Trust's overspend as it is expensive in relation to: bed occupancy; treating the infection, including having to revise operations; and potential court cases, which are not only expensive but can also seriously affect the Trust's reputation.

- It affects visitors and staff as well as patients; it involves aspects of health and safety, risk management, clinical governance, clinical audit; and it can affect all the departments in the hospital.

- Some hospital acquired infection is inevitable, because it occurs in patients whose immune systems have been weakened due to the serious nature of their illnesses or because they have been subjected to intensive medicine. However, as stated in the National Audit Office report, on average infection control teams believed a 15 per cent reduction was feasible1. Using a more cautious estimate of a 10 per cent reduction, the following case for investment was made.

How the facts were used to make the case for investment:

The Trust has about 60,000 admissions a year. If 10 per cent acquire an infection, there will be approximately 6,000 infections. If the infection delays discharge by an average 11 days and each infection costs an extra £3,000 then hospital acquired infection would be costing the hospital 66,000 bed days and £18 million. If the work of the infection control team could reduce infections by 10 per cent then the savings could be 600 infections and £1.8million. If the reduction were only 1 per cent, the cost savings would still be £180,000, equivalent to the salaries of 4-5 infection control nurses. As a result of the business case two additional infection control nurses were approved.

Source: National Audit Office Conference - Professor French, Head of Infection Control at Guy's and St Thomas' NHS Hospital and Chairman Hospital Infection Society.

Summary

The National Audit Office finding that the management of hospital acquired infection has a low profile within NHS Trusts, was echoed by a number of speakers at the National Audit Office conference. There was also general agreement that the role of the Chief Executive was crucial to improving management and control but that Chief Executives had, in the past, given the issue too little attention. However, it was generally acknowledged that the recent clinical governance and controls assurance initiatives are likely to improve strategic management input and have a positive impact on the profile and control of hospital acquired infection.

Nevertheless, a constraint on improving the management of hospital acquired infection, remains the need to ensure that sufficient resources are available for infection control. Many speakers at the National Audit Office conference supported the conclusions in the Committee of Public Accounts report that the current level of expenditure on infection control is inadequate, and that this, together with pressures from competing objectives, such as reducing waiting lists, was constraining the implementation of good infection control practices.

Summary of the main points on strengthening the strategic management of hospital acquired infection:

- there is a need to clarify lines of accountability for the infection control team within Trusts;

- the introduction of controls assurance, clinical governance and risk management should ensure that in future infection control has the profile it merits, including giving the Trust Chief Executive core responsibility for ensuring that adequate infection control arrangements are in place in the hospital;

- the Hospital Infection Control Committee needs to have a high profile within the Trust, including Board level representation and the Chief Executive or a nominated representative should be an active member of the Committee;

- the Trust's infection control programme should include all of the components of a good infection control regime and this should be reviewed regularly by the Hospital Infection Control Committee and the results reported to the Chief Executive;

- infection control resources need to be reviewed on a regular basis and benchmarked against other similar Trusts. Once it is available, staffing resources should be evaluated in the light of the assessment tool being developed by the Department and Infection Control Nurses Association; and

- a business case approach can be used to make a robust case for investing resources to improve the management and control of hospital acquired infection.

The Department's new National Patient Safety Agency[28] and the changes introduced in the Department's report "Organisation with a Memory"[29] will have important implications for the management and control of hospital acquired infection. NHS Trusts will be required to report to the new Agency those infections that are deemed to be a result of an adverse incident and which, with better management, could have been avoided. However the exact details of the reporting requirements is still under discussion. Once these have been agreed, NHS Trusts will need to consider how their current management and control arrangements compare with the reporting requirements introduced by this new initiative.

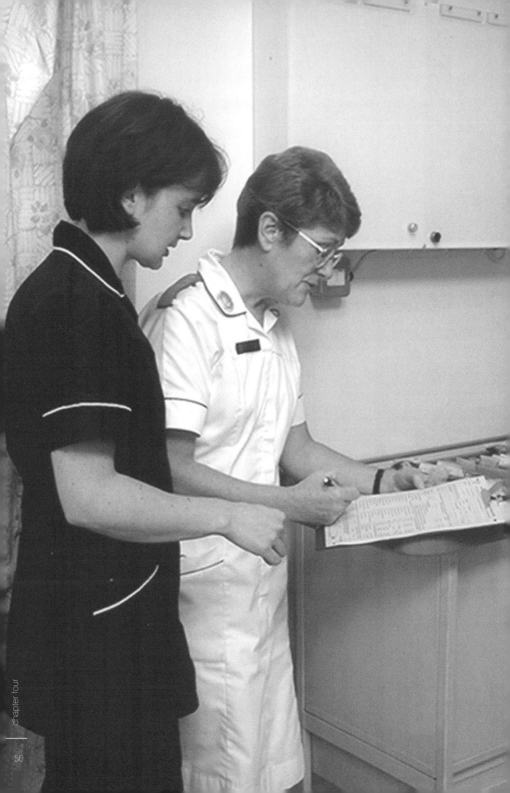

Chapter 4
Improving information and understanding

nfection control teams, senior managers and clinicians need to be well informed about the extent and costs of hospital acquired infection in their particular setting, and how this compares to the national picture. Research shows that surveillance, involving data collection, analysis and feedback of results to clinicians is central to detecting infections, dealing with them, and ultimately reducing infection rates.[1] The National Audit Office and Committee of Public Accounts reports identified surveillance as an essential component of the prevention and control of infection in hospitals.[1,7] In January 2000, the Department's programme to improve the management and control of hospital acquired infection included action needed on surveillance of hospital infection.[9] This chapter covers:

- the importance of surveillance;

- the fact that types of surveillance used and the extent to which results are fed-back to clinicians varies widely across NHS Trusts;

- how some Trusts have used local information about extent and costs to inform clinical audit activities, reduce rates of hospital acquired infection and make demonstrable cost savings;

- the development of the Nosocomial Infection National Surveillance Scheme of enhanced surveillance and the production of more robust comparative data which can be used to benchmark performance; and

- the need to develop further the national surveillance of hospital acquired infection, including the Department's decision to introduce a compulsory reporting scheme from April 2002.

The importance of surveillance

A great deal of research literature has been devoted to the importance of surveillance and the need to have clear goals for conducting surveillance. The SENIC project[19] identified that the most important purpose or goal of surveillance is to reduce the risk of acquiring a hospital infection. To achieve this goal, specific objectives for surveillance must be defined based on how the data are to be used and on the availability of financial and personnel resources for surveillance. The ultimate goal, is to obtain accurate data on infection rates which can subsequently be used to inform infection control practice and achieve a decrease in infection rates that, in turn, will reduce morbidity, mortality and treatment costs.

The Department's 1995 guidance[13] defined surveillance as the routine collection of data on infections occurring in patients and staff, its analysis and the dissemination of the results to those who need to know so that appropriate action can be taken. The main objectives were identified as:

■ the prevention and early detection of outbreaks in order to allow timely investigation and control; and

■ the assessment of infection levels over time in order to determine the need for, and measure the effect of, preventive or control measures.

Surveillance data can assist the infection control teams and Hospital Infection Control Committee when prioritising infection control activities; can aid the identification of risk factors for infection; and can reinforce the need for good practice. Surveillance should be part of the routine infection control programme and be carried out in partnership with clinical staff.[13]

The Department's 1995 guidance[13] details examples of various methods of surveillance together with their advantages and disadvantages. The guidance also draws attention to a 1992 study by Glenister et al[30] which compared selective surveillance methods against a comprehensive standard method designed to detect all infections in the population being studied. The researchers found that the best general method was laboratory based ward liaison surveillance involving clinical follow up of positive microbiology reports, plus twice-weekly visits to the wards to review other patients considered by nursing staff to have infection.[13]

The Hospital Infection Working Group recommended that the infection control team, in consultation with the Hospital Infection Control Committee, should develop a surveillance strategy which meets the needs of the hospital and takes into account areas of high risk. It should be based on:

■ continuous "alert organism" surveillance, which uses laboratory reports to identify specific micro-organisms that have the potential to cause serious disease or to spread within institutions and "alert condition" surveillance in which ward based staff have a responsibility to report specific clinical conditions such as diarrhoea to the infection control team. This surveillance should cover the whole Trust;

- pro-active continuous surveillance of microbiology specimens and laboratory results from the whole hospital to detect outbreaks or other unexpected changes in patterns of all types of infection. This requires the infection control team to scrutinise positive microbiology results on a daily basis; and

- a combination of targeted and selective surveillance in a formal programme to monitor trends in infection rates in specific groups of patients or locations in the hospital, concentrating mainly on infections that are serious in terms of morbidity, mortality and/or cost of care. The overall aim is to facilitate regular review and discussion of year on year data within the hospital.

Surveillance is used widely in NHS Trusts but the scope of surveillance and feedback of results varies

The National Audit Office found that, during 1998-1999, the majority of infection control teams carried out continuous "alert organism" surveillance.[1] Fifty-eight per cent of infection control teams carried out some form of targeted surveillance and 72 per cent selective surveillance. However, only 103 infection control teams (51 per cent of the infection control teams who carry out surveillance), produced data on infection rates and 66 per cent produced data on trends (based mainly on changes in the overall number of infections such as MRSA and *Clostridium difficile*).

The report concluded that in general surveillance needed to be done more effectively. Over 90 per cent of infection control teams had carried out some limited surveillance but there was a lack of comparable data on rates and trends. This limited NHS Trusts' ability: to have a good understanding of the infection problems, both within the Trust and in comparison with other Trusts; and to determine the effectiveness of any intervention measures employed.[1]

The Department's 1995 guidance[13] stated that: "regular feedback of surveillance to appropriate medical and nursing staff is an essential component of the surveillance process". An example, used at the conference based on an American experience illustrates the value of feedback (**Conference abstract 5**). Infection control teams are required to report these surveillance results for regular review by the Hospital Infection Control Committee and consultant in communicable disease control. The Hospital Infection Control Committee is then expected to discuss these results before sending them formally to the Trust Chief Executive. However, the National Audit Office found wide variations in feedback of surveillance data.[1]

Conference abstract 5

The importance of ensuring that data are disseminated to clinical staff

Over a prolonged period of time (1989 - 1996), the incidence of hospital acquired central venous line associated infections occurring in children admitted to the intensive care unit at a US children's hospital had been considerably higher than the US National Nosocomial Infection Surveillance Scheme (NNISS) 50th percentile. During this time surveillance data had been given to Unit Managers and Clinical Directors. In 1997, there was a change in dissemination policy. Data were reported directly to clinical staff working on the wards, with dramatic effects. They had not realised that their performance was poor compared to that at other hospitals, and a range of interventions were implemented and compliance with existing protocols enhanced. The incidence of this type of infection fell sharply to well below the 50th percentile. Since 1997 it has risen slightly but remains below the 50th percentile.

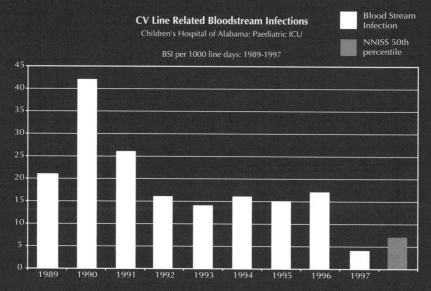

CV Line Related Bloodstream Infections
Children's Hospital of Alabama: Paediatric ICU

BSI per 1000 line days: 1989-1997

Blood Stream Infection

NNISS 50th percentile

Source: National Audit Office conference: Jennifer Wilson Senior Nurse Manager and Surveillance Co-ordinator NISU.

The benefits to be gained from spending more time on surveillance

In responding to the National Audit Office survey, a large proportion of infection control doctors and infection control nurses stated that they would like to spend less time on being reactive and more time on surveillance in order to reduce hospital acquired infection.[1] Evidence given to the House of Lords Committee on Science and Technology inquiry on antibiotic resistance made the same point.[21]

The National Audit Office report[1] noted that infection control teams were supported in their wish to spend more time on surveillance by evidence from the American SENIC project (Haley et al).[19] This comprehensive study, which involved a five year study of infection control (1970-71 to 1975-76) in over 300 hospitals, is widely regarded as the seminal piece of research into the value of surveillance of hospital acquired infection. Their results showed that those hospitals with infection control programmes which included surveillance; an infection control doctor; one infection control nurse per 250 beds; and feedback of surveillance results to clinicians, reduced infections by an average of 32 per cent. In contrast, hospitals with an infection control programme that excluded surveillance reduced rates by 6 per cent over five years, and those without effective programmes saw rates increase by 18 per cent. The research concluded that without organised routine surveillance systems, which included the feedback of results to those who need to know, even the most rigorous infection control policies are unlikely to be fully successful.

The Department's revised requirement for surveillance at NHS Trust level

The analysis of the National Audit Office survey data by the Department's regional epidemiologists included a review of the findings on surveillance. As a result of this review, the Department's action plan (HSC 2000/002) to improve the management and control of hospital infection included action to improve surveillance of hospital infection.[9] It stipulated that:

■ Chief Executives of NHS Trusts should ensure that there is appropriate staffing and information technology to undertake surveillance by 1st June 2000;

■ infection control teams should implement an appropriate programme for surveillance of infection by 1st June 2000; and

■ infection control teams should review information outputs and ensure that clinicians, managers and consultants in communicable disease control are provided with appropriate and timely information by 1st September 2000.[9]

Some infection control teams have used surveillance to reduce rates of hospital acquired infection and make demonstrable cost savings

The National Audit Office report provided details of interventions introduced as a result of surveillance, that infection control teams believed had reduced rates of hospital acquired infection and achieved demonstrable cost savings.[1] The main areas cited were in relation to MRSA and *Clostridium difficile*, particularly in the care of the elderly. Fifty-one out of 110 NHS Trusts indicated that a change in antibiotic policy had helped control *Clostridium difficile* and a similar number identified active management of MRSA including revision in antibiotic prescribing as preventing the problem (**Figure 9**).

The Nosocomial Infection National Surveillance Scheme has been an important step in the development of surveillance in the NHS

The 1995 Infection Control Working Group[13] recommended that a voluntary national reporting scheme should be established to enable hospitals to compare their data against aggregated anonymised data from other hospitals. In November 1995, following a competitive tendering exercise, the Department awarded the Public Health Laboratory Service a project to establish a national targeted surveillance scheme. The Nosocomial Infection National Surveillance Scheme (NINSS) was launched in March 1996, jointly managed and funded by the Department and Public Health Laboratory Service.[10] Participation was voluntary but the aim was that ultimately most acute hospitals would participate in the Nosocomial Infection National Surveillance Scheme. The aims of the scheme were:[1]

■ to improve patient care by assisting hospitals to change clinical practice and reduce rates and risk of hospital acquired infection; and

■ to provide national statistics on hospital acquired infection for comparison with local results.

Figure 9: How surveillance results led to changing antibiotic policy which reduced hospital acquired infections and led to demonstrable cost savings

A   Change in antibiotic policy at Scunthorpe and Goole

Concerns over increasing levels of *Clostridium difficile* associated diarrhoea in elderly patients culminated in 20 new cases in 1 ward over three days. Following an outbreak control meeting the infection control doctor developed a new antibiotic policy that recommended ceasing to use cephlasphorins on the wards and recommended suitable alternatives for different infections. To support the proposed change in policy, the infection control doctors mounted an education awareness campaign. They targeted doctors through posters in wards, giving advice on what antibiotics to use and when. As a result of this campaign and change to the antibiotic policy surveillance results showed a dramatic reduction in the rates of *Clostridium difficile* infection with the number of new cases on the Care of the Elderly ward decreasing from 163 in 1996-97 to 20 in 1997-98. It was demonstrated that the extra cost of the new antibiotic policy, estimated at £12,192 per annum, was more than offset by reducing the numbers of *Clostridium difficile* infections, estimated as around £278,000 per annum (based on associated length of stay data). There were also perceived reductions in morbidity and possibly mortality, though the full extent has not been measured.

B   Change in antibiotic policy at Addensbrookes NHS Trust

A change in the antibiotic policy at Addenbrookes NHS Trust, for the treatment of elderly patients with *Clostridium difficile*, led to a 50 per cent reduction in the number of cases of infectious diarrhoea. While acknowledging that cost savings are difficult to quantify, attempts were made to calculate savings using data calculated for the hospital and published in 1996-97. They calculated that cases of *Clostridium difficile* diarrhoea stay in hospital 20.5 days extra (39.5 days versus 19 days for controls). Based on an estimated cost of a bed of £150-£200 per day and some additional costs for diagnostic tests, antibiotics, etc, this represented an additional cost of approximately £4,000 per case of *Clostridium difficile*. The 53 fewer cases therefore represented a potential saving of 1,087 bed days (53 x 20.5 days) or £212,000 [53 x £4,000]. While this may not represent actual cost savings there is evidence that it reduced mortality, morbidity and bed occupancy.

C   Change in approach at the Norfolk and Norwich NHS Trust reduced infection rates in vascular graft patients and also saved money

The Norfolk and Norwich NHS Trust's change in its measures aimed at the control of infection in vascular graft patients led to a reduction in infection rates from 30 per cent to 12 per cent over the course of 15 months. Those due to MRSA fell from 13 per cent to 5 per cent and non MRSA from 17 per cent to 7 per cent. The costs of the change included £1,000 for change in antibiotic prophylaxis, £500 for use of pre-op wash, and £6,000 for MRSA screening. This cost increase of £7,500 compared with the estimated reduced length of stay costs of £195,000 per annum.

Source: National Audit Office report [1]

The National Audit Office[1] identified the Nosocomial Infection National Surveillance Scheme as an important infection control tool because it:

- enabled participating NHS Trusts to judge their performance against data from comparable patient groups in other hospitals;

- enabled participating NHS Trusts to work with the Nosocomial Infection National Surveillance Scheme team and others to try and make any improvements that appear to be needed;

- had the potential to develop into a truly national scheme with the scope to produce year on year data that will allow trends in hospital acquired infection in England to be monitored; and

- offered scope to adapt the methodology and results for use as a quality assessment tool, as part fulfilment of the requirements of the NHS Clinical Governance initiative.

At the conference, the National Audit Office noted that if there hadn't been a national surveillance scheme then they would have recommended that one should be established. At the time of the National Audit Office survey the Nosocomial Infection National Surveillance Scheme had been in operation for over two years, the first year of which was the pilot phase. The National Audit Office review noted that "it was still early in the life of the project" and asked whether Trusts: had experienced any benefits from participation; expected to experience any benefits in the next 2-3 years; and had experienced any difficulties participating in the scheme.

Thirty-one NHS Trusts acknowledged that they had participated in the pilot scheme and 94 NHS Trusts that they were participating in one or both modules of the scheme (relating to surgical site infections and hospital acquired bacteraemia (bloodstream) infections). Forty-two per cent of these participating Trusts said they had experienced benefits, while 44 per cent believed that they had not as yet seen the benefits. The remaining 14 per cent did not answer the question. The main benefits identified by the Trusts were the standardisation of data collection and the ability to compare results. The main problems were the time needed to collect data and the general strain on resources imposed by surveillance.[1]

The National Audit Office report noted that on balance, NHS Trusts saw the Nosocomial Infection National Surveillance Scheme as a helpful innovation. Prior to publication of the National Audit Office report in December 1999, the number of hospitals participating in one or more modules had grown to 139.[1] By June 2001, the number of hospitals that had participated in at least one surveillance period was 176; 149 had participated in surgical site infection surveillance and 93 in hospital acquired bacteraemia surveillance (66 had participated in both). In the last year, between 27 and 45 hospitals participated each quarter in the surveillance of hospital acquired bacteraemia and between 58 and 80 hospitals participated each quarter in surgical site infection surveillance (data supplied by the Nosocomial Infection Surveillance Unit at the Public Health Laboratory Service).

Surveillance results from the Nosocomial Infection National Surveillance Scheme suggest that there is scope to reduce hospital acquired infection

The National Audit Office concluded that the Nosocomial Infection National Surveillance Scheme was starting to show the benefits of surveillance. While recognising that there were some limitations to the Scheme, in particular the fact that it comprised self-selected hospitals, they considered that the data being generated provided the most comprehensive set of comparable data available to the NHS.[1] The results of the first two years' bacteraemia surveillance[31] and surgical site infection surveillance[32] were published in July 2000. These showed considerable inter-hospital variation in the incidence of hospital acquired infection which cannot be explained by case mix differences. They showed that:

■ by the end of January 2001, the National Surveillance module for Hospital Acquired Bacteraemia had analysed Patient Administration data on nearly 2 million patients.[31] This analysis identified 6,949 patients (3.5 per 1000 patient days) with one or more bacteraemias. Variations in rates occurred between specialties and between hospitals. The specialty rate for hospital acquired bacteraemia in general intensive care was 9.0 per 1000 patient days compared to 4.9 in haematology, 0.8 in general surgery (1,309 infections) and 0.5 in general medicine. There were also wide variations in rates in individual specialty groups between different hospitals. These inter-hospital variations remained after controlling for age structure and other case mix differences; and

■ the average surgical wound infection rate per 100 operations for large bowel surgery was 10.6, compared with 2.5 per 100 total hip replacement operations and 1.9 for abdominal hysterectomies.[32] These average figures conceal considerable variations in rates in patients undergoing similar procedures at different hospitals (**Figure 10**). The results strongly suggest that infection rates reflect differences in practice and that there is generally scope to reduce hospital acquired infection.

Figure 10: Results of first 44 months (to April 2001) of NINSS surgical site infection surveillance

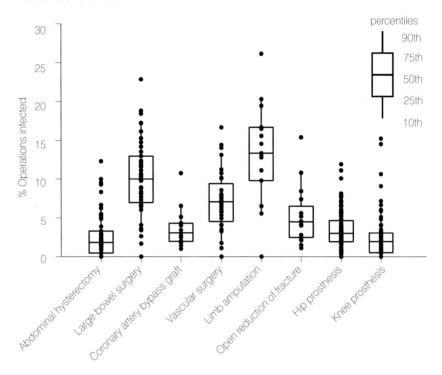

Each point in the figure represents the incidence of surgical site infection for a participating hospital. The boxes placed on the sets of points for each category give the estimates of the 25th, 50th and 75th percentiles of the incodence of surgical site infection and the ends of the verical lines represent the 10th and 90th percentiles.

Source: Public Health Laboratory Service Nosocomial Infection Surveillance Unit

While there may be valid reasons why a particular hospital is an outlier, this type of analysis allows the infection control team to investigate these reasons and to work with other hospital staff to reduce the overall extent of hospital acquired infection.[1] Jennie Wilson, speaking at the National Audit Office conference, used a specific example to illustrate this point (**Conference abstract 6**).

Conference abstract 6
Participation in NINSS can lead to a change in clinical practice

Plymouth Hospitals NHS Trust began participating in NINSS in 1997 and now carries out a systematic programme of intermittent surveillance.

Participation has led to a wide range of quality improvements in:

■ pre-operative preparation of coronary artery by-pass graft operations

■ theatre discipline

■ wound management

■ environmental cleanliness

For example: on receipt of NINSS data, orthopaedic surgeons reviewed theatre practice and identified a number of problems. They therefore revised their theatre protocols. These revisions, together with regular monitoring of surveillance data, have led to a significant reduction in infection rates.

Feedback of NINSS data has also led to an increase in the number of infection control link nurses and an overall increase in awareness of infection control principles and policies.

The overall profile of hospital acquired infection has increased with the infection control nurse being regularly asked to attend surgical audit meetings and surveillance reports being submitted to the clinical governance board.

Source: Jennifer Wilson - National Audit Office conference based on information provided by infection control nurses, Jill Swales et al, Plymouth Hospital

Ownership of surveillance results is important

Other speakers at the conference emphasised the importance of engaging clinicians in the process of data collection and spoke of the need to share the burden of data collection whilst ensuring that someone is accountable for this process (**Conference Abstract 7**). However, for this to be successful, there needs to be a thorough education programme, which would need to be repeated at regular intervals to ensure compliance with protocols and ensure new staff were aware of their responsibilities.

Some form of post-discharge surveillance is needed

The National Audit Office found that only a quarter of NHS Trusts had attempted any type of post-discharge surveillance.[1] The Committee of Pubic Accounts report recommended that post-discharge surveillance should be conducted either as part of an NHS Trust's own surveillance programme or part of the national scheme.[7] The Department's response to the Committee's report, in February 2001, noted that a UK-wide meeting of consultant microbiologists and others with a key interest in post-discharge infection was held in January 2001 to review progress and make recommendations. The new NHS Healthcare Associated Infection Surveillance Steering Group, set up in September 2000 to provide the Department with urgent recommendations on infection surveillance needs at local, regional and national level, is expected to take this work forward.[8]

The challenge - the future development of national surveillance

The publication of the National Audit Office report in February 2000[1] coincided with the end of the initial 5-year phase of the development of the Nosocomial Infection National Surveillance Scheme. The National Audit Office report noted that in preparation for this, the Department had commissioned a review to determine the best ways to expand and develop the scheme to meet local NHS trust and overall surveillance needs. Speaking at the National Audit Office conference, Professor Brian Duerden, Deputy Director of the Public Health Laboratory Service, noted that the Nosocomial Infection National Surveillance Scheme is entering a new phase. The scheme would be re-launched towards the end of year 2000 under a different name which would reflect the 'service' element. In making changes to the scheme, recognition would be given to the experience gained over the last five years, the findings of the National Audit Office report and the results of internal users surveys.

Conference abstract 7
Surveillance at the Royal Hospitals Belfast: the question of ownership

Advantages of the type of surveillance used at the Royal Hospitals Belfast:

■ It records denominators as well as numerators as each patient having a valid surgical procedure activates a surveillance form irrespective of whether the patient subsequently develops an infection.

■ It enables stratification of risks.

■ It can take less than 60 seconds to complete the form and as medical staff are actively involved in completing the form they feel ownership. Because they collect it, therefore it's theirs, therefore they want to know the results. This also encourages further involvement in the surveillance.

■ Feedback is through an annual report to the Chief Executive and Health Board and six monthly confidential reports to each surgeon. The reports utilise both statistical and visual prompts. More recently, surgeons/groups of surgeons/other medical staff have been shown the live database and allowed to interrogate it directly, in interactive sessions. As a result staff have been able to see, first hand, the versatility of the data set in addressing key questions and the value of surveillance. This has ensured that clinicians are engaged in the process and has encouraged a sense of ownership and better understanding of the results.

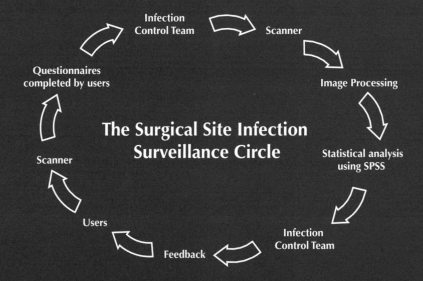

Infection Control Team → Scanner → Image Processing → Statistical analysis using SPSS → Infection Control Team → Feedback → Users → Scanner → Questionnaires completed by users → Infection Control Team

The Surgical Site Infection Surveillance Circle

The changes he anticipated included:

■ changing the emphasis so that surveillance is seen as a clinical activity that needs to be owned by those caring for patients;

■ providing local Trusts with the tools to undertake surveillance and comparative data to help inform infection control programmes;

■ doubling the Department's investment in surveillance;[8] and

■ extending coverage to obtain data for more clinical areas such as intensive care settings and on links between antimicrobial resistance and prescribing.

Evidence to the Committee of Public Accounts

The Committee of Public Accounts was concerned at the lack of robust, up-to-date, data on the extent of hospital acquired infection and found it difficult to see how the Department of Health, health authorities and NHS Trusts can target activity and resources to best effect.[7] The Department told the Committee that that they were doubling their investment in surveillance to £1 million a year. They stated that they were extending coverage to obtain data for more clinical areas, such as intensive care settings, and links between antimicrobial resistance and prescribing. They expected that the new system should generate data more systematically and in three to four years they should have very good data. As a result of this work, the Department's aim was to develop measures, targets and benchmarks that will allow people to know whether their practice was getting better.[7] The Committee welcomed these developments but recommended that the Department should go further and make surveillance mandatory.

At the Conference Dr Pat Troop, Deputy Chief Medical Officer, identified surveillance as one of the underpinning programmes of the Department's prevention and control strategy. In October 2000, the Minister of State for Health announced that surveillance of hospital acquired infection would be made compulsory for all NHS Acute Trusts from April 2001 and that data would be published from 2002.[33]

In February 2001, the Department told the Committee of Public Accounts that they had established a new Healthcare Associated Infection Surveillance Steering Group, chaired by a Trust Chief Executive, to provide urgent recommendations on infection surveillance needs at local, regional and national level.[8] It is intended that this will "build and improve on the limited coverage of the Nosocomial Infection National Surveillance Scheme, to deliver national surveillance reporting of hospital acquired infection by all Acute Trusts from 1 April 2001."

As a first step, and in the light of advice from the Steering Group, from April 2001, the Department has introduced a requirement for compulsory healthcare acquired bacteraemia surveillance.[34] Arrangements have been put in place for NHS Trusts to provide information on bacteraemia caused by methicillin resistant *Staphylococcus aureus*, and for this information to be published from April 2002. The aim is to identify those hospitals that are outliers or where there is an increasing trend so that appropriate action can be taken. A second tier of surveillance is being developed to help hospitals with that process. The Department also has work in hand to extend these reporting arrangements as soon as mechanisms can be put in place to cover other priority organisms, including surgical site infections, focussing initially on orthopaedic surgery.

Conclusions

Nationally it is known that hospital acquired infection can have serious consequences for patients and may be costing the NHS as much as £1 billion a year. It is therefore important to understand as much as possible about the extent and types of infections that are occurring at the local level. While NHS Trusts will have an irreducible minimum level of infection, it is important that they take all reasonable steps to reduce the extent of avoidable hospital acquired infection.

Surveillance of hospital acquired infection is the key to obtaining the information necessary to identify areas of concern, both locally and nationally, and to enable Trusts to target prevention activity more effectively. Surveillance data can be used as a tool to evaluate the outcome of initiatives taken and provide senior managers and clinicians with the information necessary to inform their practices and procedures. It can also provide infection control teams with relevant information to enable them to make an effective case for investing in infection control. The overall impact of better information is that the Department and NHS Trusts will have a better grip on the extent and cost of the problem which should benefit patients, staff and the health service more generally.

The Nosocomial Infection National Surveillance Scheme showed the value of enhanced targeted surveillance and how this can be used to identify outliers and to work with individual Trusts, and within Trusts with individual clinicians, to reduce infection rates. The decision to develop a new, more comprehensive scheme which builds on and improves the limited coverage of the current Nosocomial Infection National Surveillance Scheme is therefore welcomed.

The key points that arise from this review of surveillance are:

At the national level

There is a need for the Department to determine as soon as possible the extent and coverage of their new enhanced surveillance scheme and the extent to which the information from this will be published as part of the new compulsory national surveillance reporting system.[8]

The requirement for each hospital to publish the numbers of bacteraemia infections, which will be used as a marker for infection control practice and for the prevalence of MRSA, is a positive development but will need to be monitored closely to ensure consistency of reporting, both within and between Regions.

Consideration will also need to be given to the extent to which the new surveillance system meets the concerns raised by the Committee of Public Accounts.

At NHS Trusts level

Appropriate surveillance systems need to be established. These will need to conform to the new national requirements for surveillance and also:

■ use nationally comparable definitions;

■ include continuous alert organism and alert condition laboratory based reporting;

■ involve an agreed form of targeted surveillance, to generate rates and trend data;

■ have some method for collecting information on post-discharge infections;

■ link to antibiotic prescribing;

■ facilitate comparison of local results with the national picture; and

■ have appropriate mechanisms for efficient feedback of surveillance results.

There will also be a need to ensure that there is appropriate staffing and IT support to undertake this surveillance.[9]

Chapter 5

Reducing hospital acquired infection by influencing clinical practice

The National Audit Office report acknowledged that while not all hospital acquired infection can be prevented there is much that can be done to reduce infection rates.[1] Indeed, the Department of Health when publishing their new evidence based guidelines in January 2001[35] stated that:

"Not all hospital acquired infection is avoidable but a significant proportion is preventable. Better application of existing knowledge and adherence to good practice can make a major difference." Professor Liam Donaldson, Chief Medical Officer and Sarah Mullaly, Chief Nursing Officer - letter accompanying publication of Department Commissioned Guidelines for the Prevention and Control of Hospital Acquired Infection - January 2001.

As noted in chapter 2, on average infection control teams believe that, up to 15 per cent of hospital acquired infection could be prevented by better application of existing knowledge and realistic infection control policies (estimate based on a bed weighted average of responses from 174 infection control teams). The Nosocomial Infection National Surveillance Scheme data in chapter 4 show wide variations in infection rates between the same specialties in different hospitals, which suggests that there is significant scope to reduce infection rates. This chapter looks at the different preventative activities that may contribute towards a reduction in rates and also improve overall management and control. It details the types of preventative action that all staff, patients and visitors need to be aware of and focuses on factors identified in the National Audit Office report and conference as being key to improving the effectiveness of infection control activities at the level of patient care. In particular, it focuses on the following assertions:

■ hospital acquired infection prevention and control are everyone's responsibility;

■ healthcare workers need more knowledge about infection control;

■ there is a lack of compliance with infection control procedures, for example hand-hygiene;

- the state of hospital environmental cleanliness impacts on the effectiveness of infection control;

- prudent use of antibiotics and monitoring of resistance is essential; and

- whilst intervention activities such as isolation and screening for MRSA are used, not enough is known about their effectiveness.

Hospital acquired infection is everyone's responsibility

The Department's guidance, in particular the controls assurance standards, clearly signifies that infection prevention and control is not just the responsibility of those specifically employed to combat microbial risk.[12,13] All health care workers have a responsibility for adopting good infection prevention and control practices.[21] John Denham MP, the then Minister of State for Health, when launching the Department's new Antibiotic Strategy at the National Audit Office conference in June 2000, stated that:

"Infection control is of course an old problem but one that we now face in new and sometimes frightening forms, including the 'super bugs' as referred to in the tabloid newspapers. And everyone in the NHS, from the Trust Chief Executive to senior consultants, to nurses and ancillary staff, has a role to play in modernising the fight against hospital acquired infection."

The views of other speakers at the National Audit Office conference endorsed these sentiments (**Conference abstract 8**).

Conference abstract 8
Synopsis of views from speakers at the National Audit Office Conference on the need for everyone to accept responsibility for prevention

Graham Elderfield, Chief Executive Isle of Wight Healthcare NHS Trust - "Good infection control cannot be done by just one or two infection control nurses. It requires an effective team right across the hospital of doctors, nurses and managers working together."

A system of link nurses can help increase awareness of infection control issues

A number of NHS Trusts have adopted a system of 'link nurses' to help increase awareness of infection control issues and assist in the early detection of outbreaks of infection.[1] Link nurses are not a substitute for the infection control nurse but are ward based staff who can help take on some of the responsibilities by acting under the direct supervision of the infection control nurse. The infection control team provides them with regular and appropriate training in infection control, which they then apply in the ward setting. In some cases they are also trained to collect surveillance data for the infection control team. To be effective, link nurses need to have sufficient clinical experience and standing to have authority with managers and colleagues.

The National Audit Office found that some 59 per cent of NHS Trusts had introduced a link nurse scheme. While link nurses can represent a valuable link between infection control nurses and nurses working at ward level, the success of these schemes varied between Trusts.[1] Fifty per cent of NHS Trusts who used the scheme reported that they found it to be fairly successful in improving infection control and 20 per cent found it very successful, with 18 per cent considering it fairly unsuccessful. At the National Audit Office conference Susan Macqueen, the then Chair of the Infection Control Nurses Association, referred to a study that found compliance with infection control standards was higher when link nurses were present on the ward (Millward et al).[36] She cited high staff turnover, as one factor that makes it difficult to ensure that link nurses are provided with sufficient training in infection control issues. The appointment of junior staff, who lack the experience and authority needed to be an effective link nurse, was a further explanation for unsuccessful schemes. She agreed with the findings in the National Audit Office report that link nurse schemes may not be appropriate for all NHS Trusts, particularly large Trusts with multiple sites and high staff turnover.[1] **Conference abstract 9 overleaf**, illustrates how one NHS Trust has implemented a successful link nurse scheme.

Dr Louise Teare, Consultant Microbiologist Mid-Essex Hospitals NHS Trust - "Infection control is everyone's business - and must be owned by everyone involved in health care."

Professor Gary French, Chairman Hospital Infection Society - "Hospital acquired infection is everybody's problem, it's not just the job of the infection control doctor and infection control nurse to stop infections, it's the job of everyone working in the Trust."

Conference abstract 9
The development of an infection control link nurse programme

The infection control team was concerned that the profile of infection control was not particularly high, with responsibility placed solely on one infection control doctor and one infection control nurse in a 860 bed NHS Trust. The infection control team convinced the NHS Trust that better infection control and feedback to clinicians could reduce infection rates and save costs.

The NHS Trust agreed to develop an infection control link nurse programme, which would be introduced over 4 years in 3 phases: setting up and establishing; ward standard setting; and management ownership. Each ward and department was asked to nominate a link nurse and deputy, who became part of the Infection Control Liaison Group - a total of 57 link nurses. These nurses are readily identifiable to ward staff and have regular contact with the infection control team including 3-monthly formal training sessions. Their main responsibilities are education and surveillance. The NHS Trust has recognised the importance of link nurses by awarding them formal contracts.

The link nurse programme has raised the profile of infection control. The infection control team has been incorporated into the risk management group at NHS Trust level giving Infection control a high status and authority. Their knowledge base and the reliability and coverage of surveillance has increased significantly and there is evidence that this is helping to deliver substantial gains in performance; and provide a reduction in hospital acquired infection, length of stay, drug costs and so on.

Source: Conference Presentation by Dr Louise Teare Consultant Microbiologist at the Mid-Essex Hospital Services NHS Trust

Healthcare workers need more knowledge about good infection control practices

The Department's 1995 guidance on the management of hospital acquired infection identified education as a key component of an effective infection control programme and advocated that infection control teams should provide an education programme for all hospital employees and students.[13] The National Audit Office found[1] that this was not necessarily happening. For example:

■ ten per cent of NHS Trusts did not provide induction training for nurses and nursing assistants;

■ seventeen per cent of NHS Trusts failed to provide induction training for junior doctors;

■ a worrying 97 per cent did not provide induction training for senior doctors; and

■ only 59 per cent of NHS Trusts provided induction training for food handlers and 68 per cent for cleaners.

The National Audit Office also found that the annual update training was not as thorough as it should be: only 63 per cent of infection control teams provided annual update training for nurses, 47 per cent for health care assistants and 12 per cent for senior doctors.[1]

The results of a Scottish survey in 1999, which looked at the amount of infection control education healthcare professionals received, showed a similar picture. On average qualified nurses received 2.5 minutes of infection control education; paramedics allied to medicine received 3 minutes; junior doctors, 2.2 minutes; and other sectors 0.6 minutes.[37] Graham Elderfield, Chief Executive of the Isle of White NHS Trust, told the National Audit Office Conference that "the ignorance of hospital staff in relation to infection control issues was the biggest challenge facing his infection control nurse."

Infection control teams' ability to deliver training is limited by the amount of time they have available to run the training courses and staff finding the time to attend[1]. Some NHS Trusts, however, have developed computer assisted learning packages to help improve staff awareness. A number of bespoke systems are also available, including a system developed by King's College Hospital, London, entitled 'Introduction to Infection Control'.[1] The Infection Control Nurses Association are also in the process of developing a computer assisted learning package aimed at all grades of staff.[7]

chapter five

Some education and training in infection control is provided as part of the undergraduate medical and health professional training courses.[7] However, the House of Lords Select Committee of Science and Technology report on antibiotic resistance (1998),[21] found that coverage of infection control in health professional training courses was limited. They recommended changes to the curricula of professional education for doctors and nurses to give more time to the study of appropriate prescribing and infection control. Progress on improving the infection control element in medical education has been slow but, in April 2001, the Department and the British Society of Antimicrobial Chemotherapy were engaged in developing some educational materials. The Department have also raised the matter with the General Medical Council in the context of the review of "Tomorrow's Doctors", the framework document for medical education.[38]

Speaking at the conference, Susan Macqueen noted that the Infection Control Nurses Association has asked the English National Board for Nursing, Midwifery and Health Visiting to place more emphasis on infection control in their current review of the curriculum for undergraduate nurses. In 1999 a new model for nurse education and training was launched following publication of the Department's nursing strategy "Making a Difference"[39] and the "Fitness for Practice" report issued by the United Kingdom Central Council for Nursing, Midwifery and Health Visiting Commission for Education.[40] These include an increased emphasis on practical skills and an education system that is more responsive to the needs of the NHS. In response, the Infection Control Nurses Association, produced a paper on standards for pre-registration infection control education which has been submitted to the National Boards for Nursing, Midwifery and Health Visiting and individual higher education institutions. They are also producing a consensus document on professional competencies for infection control.

Infection control policies need to be easily available and regularly updated

The Department's 1995 guidance[13] indicated that infection control teams should provide written, easily accessible, up-to-date information on infection control procedures and arrangements. However, the National Audit Office found that compliance with this requirement was poor.[1] While the majority of Trusts had combined their policies and procedures in an infection control manual (95 per cent of Trusts had their own manual, with only 8 per cent failing to be updated in the last 4 years) they were not readily accessible to staff. The Department have accepted the recommendation in the National Audit Office report and are looking at developing a single Infection Control Manual, which builds on the one issued in Scotland.[8]

Access to up-to-date information on policies and procedures can be facilitated by the appropriate use of information technology. For example, infection control manuals have been converted into electronic format, enabling clinical staff to access information 24 hours a day at the click of a button. This also allows infection control practitioners access to up-to-date polices and practices with relative ease and at relatively low cost. Access can be facilitated further by the use of interactive computer packages.[1] The NHS Plan Implementation Programme intends that all NHS staff will have basic common desktop and NHSnet connection by March 2003.[6] This should improve the scope for using IT to disseminate infection control policies and procedures.[8]

Evidence based guidelines are important, in that they provide assurance and help improve practice

Infection control teams noted that the lack of evidence based guidelines (particularly the need for evidence of what works and why) was a constraint to ensuring compliance with good infection control policies, and persuading staff more readily to adopt or change practices.[4] In January 2001, the Department published new evidence based guidelines for the prevention and control of hospital acquired infection, as a supplement to the Journal of Hospital Infection.[35] The Department commissioned these guidelines from Thames Valley University in March 1998. They cover various elements of clinical practice for preventing the spread of hospital acquired infection, including multi-drug resistant organisms. The guidelines are comprised of three components:

■ general principles for preventing infections in hospitals including environmental cleanliness and hand hygiene practices;

■ the prevention of hospital acquired infections associated with the use of central venous catheters; and

■ the prevention of hospital acquired infections associated with the use of short-term in-dwelling urethral catheters.

In publishing the guidelines the Department declared that their intention was that they should inform the development of detailed operational protocols at NHS Trust level, and may be used to ensure that these protocols cover the most important principles for preventing hospital acquired infection. The guidelines have been distributed to a range of health care professionals, including infection control nurses, infection control doctors and clinical governance leads. The guidelines are expected to be used as an audit tool of clinical practice and be incorporated into local clinical governance programmes. In publishing the guidelines the Chief

Medical Officer and Chief Nursing Officer stated that "All of the recommendations are endorsed equally and none are regarded as optional".[35]

There is a lack of compliance with effective infection control strategies - the example of hand hygiene

Effective hand hygiene is possibly the most important factor in preventing hospital acquired infection but compliance is poor. Most infection control teams have run hand-washing campaigns but while there was usually an immediate improvement, the impact was reduced within a short time.[1]

In March 1999, in recognition of the problems with hand hygiene, a Handwashing Liaison Group (comprising the Hospital Infection Society, Association of Medical Microbiologists, Department of Health, Infection Control Nurses Association, Royal College of Nursing Midwifery and Health Visiting and Public Health Laboratory Service) issued an action plan on handwashing.[41] The Department sent this document to all NHS Chief Executives, public health directors and microbiologists in England.[1]

The action plan[41] was strongly supported by the National Audit Office.[1] It highlights the Chief Executives' responsibilities in relation to infection control. It calls for:

■   the introduction or re-introduction of hand hygiene policies and standards;

■   the development of model wards and good role models, which are supported by Chief Executives; and

■   the evaluation of compliance with Trust policies and infection rates over time.

Given the evidence of poor compliance identified in the National Audit Office survey, the strong views expressed about the importance of hand hygiene and lack of compliance, the National Audit Office strongly endorsed this initiative and the recommendations of the Handwashing Liaison Group.[1]

The Committee of Public Accounts viewed the poor compliance with guidance on hand hygiene as inexcusable.[7] The Department told the Committee that the Controls Assurance Standards on Infection Control require NHS Trusts to have a policy on hand hygiene and to provide education and training in this area. These measures are to be reviewed by internal audit as part of the new NHS performance management process.[8] These arrangements are also open to review by the

Commission for Health Improvement and the Audit Commission. The Department drew attention to the fact that the new evidence based guidelines, issued in January 2001, include 7 recommendations on hand hygiene[35] (**Figure 11**). The Department agreed to audit progress and report back to the Committee by the end of 2001.

Figure 11: Recommendations arising from a review of all available evidence concerning hand hygiene practice - Department of Health commissioned guidelines

All recommendations are endorsed equally and none is regarded as optional:

■ Hands must be decontaminated immediately before each and every episode of direct patient contact/care and after any activity that potentially results in hands becoming contaminated.

■ Hands that are visibly soiled or potentially grossly contaminated with dirt or organic material must be washed with liquid soap and water.

■ Apply an alcohol based rub or wash hands with liquid soap and water to decontaminate hands between caring for different patients or between different caring activities for the same patient.

■ Remove all wrist and ideally hand jewellery at the beginning of each clinical shift before regular hand decontamination begins. Cuts and abrasions must be covered with waterproof dressing.

■ Effective handwashing techniques involve three stages: preparation, washing and rinsing, and drying. Preparation requires wetting hands under tepid running water before applying liquid soap or an antimicrobial preparation. The handwash solution must come into contact with all the surfaces of the hand. The hands must be rubbed together vigorously for a minimum of 10-15 seconds, paying particular attention to the tips of the fingers, the thumbs and the areas between fingers. Hands should be rinsed thoroughly prior to drying with good quality paper towels.

■ When decontaminating hands using an alcohol handrub, hands should be free of dirt and organic material. The handrub solution must come into contact with all the surfaces of the hand. The hands must be rubbed together vigorously, paying particular attention to the tips of the fingers, the thumbs and the areas between fingers, and until the solution has evaporated and hands are dry.

■ Apply an emollient hand cream regularly to protect skin from the drying effects of regular hand decontamination. If a particular soap or antimicrobial handwash or alcohol product causes skin irritation, seek occupational health advice.

Source: The Journal of Hospital Infection - Supplement, January 2001 - EPIC Guidelines Development Team National Evidence Based Guidelines for preventing healthcare associated infections:[35] standard principles.

chapter two

Poor compliance with hospital environmental cleanliness standards impacts on infection control

Departmental guidance requires infection control teams to collaborate with other relevant staff in monitoring the implementation and effectiveness of the hospital's routine procedures on environmental cleanliness. The aim of this monitoring is to help prevent hospital acquired infection.[9]

Evidence to the House of Lords inquiry in autumn 1998[21] strongly supported the view that standards in hospital hygiene were slipping. Poor hygiene was implicated in some outbreaks of hospital infection and the Infection Control Nurses Association was especially concerned about cleaning of hospital wards. The Select Committee recommended that infection control and basic hygiene should be at the heart of good hospital practice.

Following the House of Lords Select Committee report Resistance to Antibiotics and other Anti-microbial Agents,[21] the Department issued HSC 1999/049[42] detailing action for NHS Trusts and health authorities, requiring them to "put infection control and basic hygiene where they belong at the heart of good management and clinical practice with appropriate resources."

In 1999, the Infection Control Nurses Association in collaboration with the Association of Domestic Managers developed a set of national cleaning standards.[43] The aims of the standards were to:

■ raise the profile of environmental cleanliness;

■ develop an audit tool for measuring standards of environmental cleanliness; and

■ develop recommendations concerning the provision of domestic services.

In May 2000, following publication of the National Audit Office report[1] and concerns raised at the Committee of Public Accounts hearing[7] about evidence of poor hygiene, the Health Secretary, Alan Milburn MP, re-issued the "Standards for Environmental Cleanliness in Hospitals" for implementation by all NHS Trusts.[44] The aim was that the standards document should be used as an evaluation tool to assess cleaning services. Since the re-launch, a number of initiatives have served to keep hospital environmental cleanliness clearly in the media spotlight.

For example:

■ In July 2000, as part of the NHS Plan,[45] the Health Minister Lord Hunt launched a new NHS "Hospital Clean-Up" initiative[46] to improve hospital cleanliness and patients' experience of their local hospital. Eight NHS Trusts were chosen to spearhead the drive to clean up NHS hospitals and act as models of good practice. In addition, £31 million was allocated directly to NHS Trusts in 2000-2001 to secure improvements in the patient's environment, including levels of hygiene and cleanliness and a further £30 million earmarked for 2001-2002. NHS Trusts are expected to allocate personal responsibility for monitoring cleanliness around the hospital to a member of their Trust Board.[7]

■ In October 2000, the Minister announced that every hospital would have unannounced inspection visits by specialist inspection teams to evaluate the standards of cleanliness with the results available to the local press.[47] At the same time he announced that the NHS would no longer have to cut costs by compulsory market testing of services such as catering and cleaning. This was linked to the need for a more flexible and less dogmatic approach to cleaning.

■ The results of the first series of inspections in November 2000 showed a significant number of hospitals failed to achieve acceptable standards and they attracted a great deal of adverse publicity.[48]

■ In December 2000, the NHS Plan Implementation Programme included the following targets:[6]

  - by April 2002, all hospitals should have senior sisters and charge nurses in place who must be given the necessary resources to sort out the fundamentals of care in the form of a ward environment budget (worth a minimum of £5000 in 2001-2002);

  - from April 2001, all hospitals need to invest to meet standards of cleanliness set out in their Cleanliness Action Plan and all need to routinely monitor patients' views on the cleanliness of hospitals. National standards of cleanliness are to form part of the Performance Assessment Framework against which every hospital will be measured; and

  - by June 2001, all hospitals were to have a plan, supported by sufficient resources, to introduce ward housekeepers. Hospitals should have introduced such services by December 2004.

chapter five

■ In January 2001, the Health Minister announced that Ward Sisters would be given a new role in enforcing standards of cleanliness throughout NHS hospitals. Also, that from April 2002, 500 Matrons are expected to be back on the wards to ensure the National Hospital Cleaning Standards are met and maintained. They will be accountable for a group of wards, and should be easily identifiable, highly visible, accessible and authoritative figures. They have the power to halt payments to cleaning contractors if they fail to meet standards.[49]

■ The Department's new evidence based guidelines,[35] published in January 2001, included the following environmental cleanliness guidelines based on action recommended in the NHS Plan:[45]

- the hospital environment must be visibly clean, free from dust and soilage, and acceptable to patients, their visitors and staff;

- where a piece of equipment is used for more than one patient, for example a commode or bath hoist, it must be cleaned following each and every episode of use;

- statutory requirements must be met in relation to the safe disposal of clinical waste, laundry arrangements for used and infected linen, food hygiene and pest control; and

- all staff involved in hospital hygiene activities must be included in education and training related to the prevention of hospital acquired infection.

■ In March 2001, details of the above initiatives and the National Audit Office and Committee of Public Accounts Reports were presented to the House of Lords Select Committee's follow up review to their report on Resistance to Antibiotics. The Select Committee's subsequent report[38] warmly welcomed these initiatives and the declaration by the Parliamentary Under Secretary of State for Health, Yvette Cooper MP, that infection control and basic hygiene are core issues for the NHS.

■ In April 2001, the results of the second series of inspection visits were announced. These show a marked improvement in cleaning standards although media coverage still tends to focus on continuing problems (**Figure 12**).[49]

	Red (poor)	Yellow (acceptable)	Green (excellent)
Autumn 2000	253	298	162
April 2001	42	367	280

Source: Results of the independent unannounced inspections[49] showing the numbers of hospitals in each category.

Prudent use of antibiotics and other antimicrobials is essential

Antibiotic resistance is a growing problem

Antibiotics, discovered in the late 1930s, were seen as the magic bullet designed to treat all infections. Their discovery led to safer medical and surgical practice and prolongation of life expectancy. Indeed, antibiotics have been used successfully for more than 50 years to treat and control bacterial infections. While antibiotics have proved useful in the treatment of infection, their use has led to the emergence of highly resistant strains of bacteria such as methicillin resistant *Staphyloccus aureus* (MRSA) and vancomycin resistant *Enterococci* (VRE) resistant to more than one antimicrobial. In some very rare cases bacteria have emerged that are resistant to all antimicrobials. A number of reports have documented the situation.[3,21,38,50,51,52,53] These drug resistant infections are more common in hospitals where high levels of antibiotic usage allow organisms to evolve; and the close concentration of people with increased susceptibility to infection allows the organisms to spread.[13]

A significant milestone in highlighting concerns about antibiotic resistance was the House of Lords Select Committee on Science and Technology Inquiry into Resistance to Antibiotics and other Antimicrobial Agents, conducted in 1998.[21] The Committee reported that:

"This enquiry has been an alarming experience which leaves us convinced that resistance to antibiotics and other anti-effective agents constitutes a major threat to public health and ought to be recognised as such more widely than it is at present."

chapter five

At the National Audit Office conference, Lord Soulsby, Chairman of the House of Lords Select Committee on Science and Technology Inquiry,[21] illustrated the significance of the problem. He provided examples of antibiotics whose therapeutic action has either been lost or is threatened and the common diseases and organisms that they were designed to target (**Figure 13**). He noted that no new classes of antibiotics have reached the market in the last 25 years, and no new ones were anticipated over the next 5-10 years (although there is at least one in the early stages of development and another in the late stage of development). He described the present position as a "desperate situation."

Figure 13: Examples of valuable therapies now lost or imperilled by the spread of resistance

Organism	Disease	Agents lost or threatened
Pneumococcus	Pneumonia, otitis, meningitis	Penicillin, many others
Meningococcus	Meningitis, septicaemia	Sulphonamides, (penicillin)
Haemophilus influenzae	Meningitis	Ampicillin, chloramphenicol
Staphylococcus aureus	Wound infection, sepsis	Penicillin, Penicillinase-resistant penicillins, other agents
Salmonella typhi	Typhoid fever	Most relevant agents
Shigella spp	Bacillary dysentry	Most relevant agents
Gonococcus	Gonorrhoea	Sulphonamides, penicillin, tetracycline, (ciprofloxacin)
Plasmodium falciparum	Severe malaria	Chloroquine, pyrimethamine, (mefloquine, quinine)
Escherichia coli (coliforms)	Urinary infection, septicaemia	Ampicillin, trimethoprim, others

Source: Conference Presentation by Lord Soulsby of Swaffam Prior

Inappropriate prescribing is a key factor in the development of resistance. This includes inappropriate use of antibiotics for self-limiting or viral infections such as colds, and some sore throats and, where antibiotics are justified, an inappropriate drug and/or treatment regime selected. Whilst in the UK the use of antibiotics is conservative compared to that in other countries, witnesses to the Select Committee on Science and Technology indicated that between 5-50 per cent of antibiotic prescriptions are inappropriate, the proportion varying with geographical location.[21] Speaking at the National Audit Office conference, Dr Geoff Scott, Consultant Microbiologist at the University College London Hospitals NHS Trust, commented that in one London suburb the number of antibiotic prescriptions issued by GPs varied from zero to 2,165 per 1,000 in an age adjusted population. The availability of antibiotics over the counter in some countries also contributes to the situation, as does the failure of patients to complete a full course of antibiotics.

There is also evidence that inappropriate use of antibiotics in animal husbandry, in particular the use of antibiotics in low quantities as growth promoters may result in antimicrobial resistance being transferred directly from animals to humans via the food chain.[21] **Figure 14** illustrates the mechanisms that give rise to antibiotic resistance and describes how such resistance may arise.

Slowing the rise of antibiotic resistance

The Government's response to the Select Committee on Science and Technology Inquiry into Resistance to Antibiotics and other Antimicrobial Agents report was issued on 17 December 1998.[52] The Government welcomed the Select Committee's report and stated its commitment to addressing antimicrobial resistance, including outlining a number of initiatives underway or planned. The Government's strategy to address antimicrobial resistance was based on three key elements: infection control, prudent antimicrobial use and surveillance.

Figure 14: How antibiotic resistance arises

The development of antibiotic resistance

- Antimicrobial resistance may be innate or acquired. Innate resistance refers to bacteria inherently resistant to one or more antibiotics. Many of these bacteria do not represent a threat to healthy humans, but may give rise to infection in hospitalised patients. Examples include the *Pseudomonas* species and some *Enterococci*.

- Acquired resistance may develop as a result of mutations in a small proportion of a bacterial population. In the presence of the antibiotic to which it is resistant, the proportion of these altered bacteria multiply and become more dominant. For example, some *Mycobacterium tuberculosis* are naturally resistant to streptomycin. In the presence of this antibiotic these bacteria soon become dominant in a population.

- Acquired resistance may also develop through the transfer of genetic material encoding resistance from one type of bacteria to another. This can occur through the direct transfer of genetic material on plasmids, on a bacterial virus or a bacteriophage, or via the direct transfer of DNA. As before in the presence of antibiotics, the susceptible bacteria are killed, thereby selecting out resistant strains which subsequently become more dominant in the population.

Antibiotic Resistance

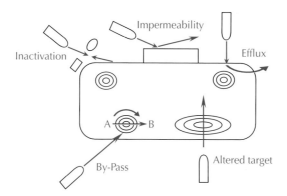

- More specifically antibiotic resistance develops through a variety of molecular mechanisms that pathogens have developed to circumvent antimicrobials.

The mechanisms that give rise to antibiotic resistance

1   Inactivation - the bacteria inactivate the drug before it reaches its target within the bacterial cell.

2   Impermeability - the outer layers of the cell are impermeable preventing the drug from entering the cell.

3   Alteration of target site - the target is altered so that it is no longer recognised by the antibiotic.

4   Efflux - the drug enters the bacteria but is then pumped out.

5   By-pass - the bacteria acquire an alternative metabolic pathway resulting in the antibiotic's target being made redundant.

Source: Conference Presentation Lord Soulsby

The Department's action for the NHS, following the Government's response to the House of Lords Select Committee report included the following goals:[42]

■ to minimise morbidity and mortality due to antimicrobial resistant infection, including hospital acquired infection;

■ to contribute to the control of antimicrobial resistant organisms; and

■ to this end, facilitate more efficient and effective use of NHS resources.

This was to be achieved through:

■ strengthening prevention and control of communicable disease, including infection control;

■ optimising antimicrobial prescribing; and

■ improving surveillance of communicable disease and infection caused by antimicrobial resistant organisms and monitoring antimicrobial usage to provide the information base for action.

A number of other reports and documents have called for the prudent use of antimicrobials in clinical practice, veterinary practice, animal husbandry, agriculture and horticulture, this being viewed as paramount to slowing the rise of resistance.[51,53] Speaking at the conference, Dr Geoff Scott advocated a pragmatic approach to antibiotic prescribing policies:

■ forbid certain antibiotics;

■ restrict prophylaxis to a single dose;

■ rotate antibiotics (although Dr Scott acknowledged that he was unaware of any good data that demonstrated that this has a significant effect on resistance); and

■ operate an antibiotic stop policy, requiring pharmacies to question whether they still need to give antibiotics after a set number of days.

The UK Strategy

The UK strategy for tackling the rise of antimicrobial resistance,[3] was launched at the National Audit Office conference in June 2000 by the Health Minister. This strategy is the result of successful collaboration between England, Scotland, Wales and Northern Ireland and, again, consists of the three inter-related elements: surveillance; prudent antimicrobial use; and infection control (**Figure 15**).

Figure 15: The UK Antimicrobial Resistance Strategy and Action Plan.

The three key inter-related elements of the UK strategy are:

- **Surveillance:** the establishment and maintenance of surveillance systems to monitor the problem over time, evaluate practice, and provide data on resistant organisms, illness due to them and antimicrobial usage necessary to inform action.

- **Prudent antimicrobial use:** to reduce unnecessary and inappropriate exposure of micro-organisms to antimicrobial agents and similar drugs in clinical practice, veterinary practice, animal husbandry, agriculture and horticulture and to develop an information campaign to educate the public as to why antibiotics need to be used more carefully.

- **Infection control:** to reduce the spread of infection in general (and thus some of the need for antimicrobial agents) and of antimicrobial resistant micro-organisms in particular.

These elements need to be supported by the provision of education, communication, research organisational support, appropriate information technology, and where necessary legislation and regulation.

To be effective, a co-ordinated approach is required at international and national level, and at the level of individual NHS Trusts.

Source: The UK Antimicrobial Resistance Strategy and Action Plan[3]

The Committee of Public Accounts highlighted their concerns about the growth of antibiotic resistance[7] but welcomed the Department's actions, including the new UK strategy to tackle antibiotic resistant infections.[3] The Committee recommended that this work should lead to evidence-based guidance on effective prescribing strategies.[7] The Department noted that the problem of antibiotic resistance is constantly changing and that the current strategy, which is intended to cover the next three years, will be kept under constant review and evolve with time to take account of changes in resistance patterns, scientific advances and organisational changes.[8] They advised the Committee of Public Accounts that the Interdepartmental Steering Group is undertaking this work, with advice from an expert Specialist Advisory Committee on Antimicrobial Resistance.

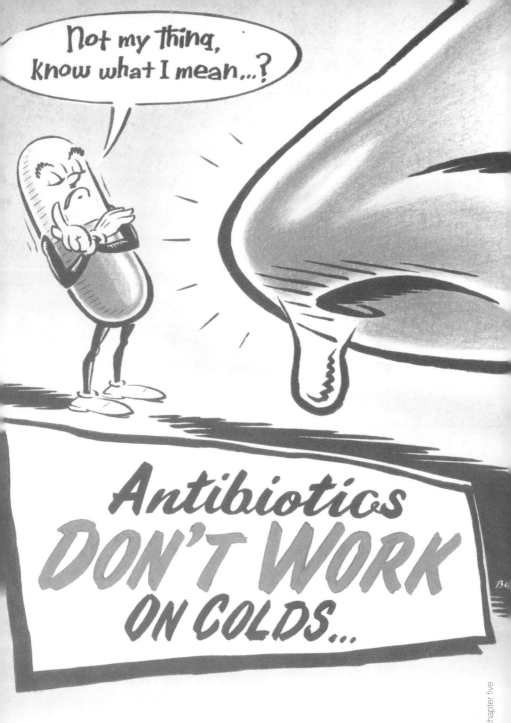

NHS

Department of Health

Since publication of the UK Strategy,[3] two further initiatives have been launched:[8]

■ a Clinical Prescribing Sub Group, set up by the Interdepartmental Steering Group, is looking at ways of optimising and monitoring prescribing of antimicrobials in clinical practice, through professional education, promotion of evidence based guidelines, prescribing organisational support and surveillance. As part of this, the Public Health Laboratory Service has developed and distributed a template which should be used as the basis of evidence-based antimicrobial prescribing policies in primary care; and

■ a clinical audit toolkit for antimicrobial prescribing and monitoring developed by the National Prescribing Centre, has been disseminated to all health authorities, Primary Care Groups/Trusts and Hospital Trusts. The National Prescribing Centre has also recruited 19 senior prescribing advisers who will be running seminars for GPs and pharmacists.

The House of Lords Science and Technology Select Committee's third report on Resistance to Antibiotics, published in March 2001,[38] noted improvements in GP prescribing (80 per cent of prescribing is in the community and antibiotic prescriptions were down by 19 per cent between September 1997 and September 1999). They believe that this had been helped, in part, by the use of non-prescription forms (forms given to patients to explain their treatment but which are not prescriptions) and also the Government's major advertising campaign (example of NHS poster is reproduced on page 85 by kind permission of the Department of Health). Both of these initiatives were principal recommendations in their 1998 Inquiry.[21]

There is a need to improve surveillance in order to obtain more robust information on antibiotic prescribing and antibiotic resistance

The Public Health Laboratory Service laboratories identify resistant organisms, both to inform treatment of particular patients and to map and monitor the rise and spread of resistance. At the time of publishing the National Audit Office report,[1] in February 2000, the Public Health Laboratory Service was developing a national Antibiotic Resistance Surveillance Programme to provide comparative data on resistance, including resistance in hospital acquired infections, at local, regional and national levels. The aim was to link these data to patterns of prescribing in hospitals and primary care. The first results of the pilot phase in the Trent region were reported to the Public Health Laboratory Service in December 1999 and this work is currently being carried forward.

The Department and Public Health Laboratory Service were also considering whether the collection of data on antibiotic prescribing could be incorporated into the national surveillance scheme. The National Audit Office report noted that the Nosocomial Infection National Surveillance Scheme collects data on the causative pathogens and as such provides some information on antibiotic resistance in hospital acquired infection, for example the surgical site infections caused by MRSA as a proportion of all staphylococcal infections.[1]

The House of Lords Science and Technology Select Committee's third report on Resistance to Antibiotics, published in March 2001[38] recognised that surveillance and data collection are crucial in the fight against resistance. However, they were concerned that this has continued to be hampered by the existence of incompatible systems of information technology. Overall they were encouraged at the tangible progress that has been made, particularly in bringing down levels of use of antibiotics in both humans and animals. The Committee concluded however that there was much more still to do, particularly in bearing down on MRSA and other resistant infections in hospitals and community settings, and in bridging gaps and incompatibilities in surveillance.

There is a need for more information on the effectiveness of intervention activities

Isolation is an expensive but effective form of infection control but facilities are limited

The Department's 1995 guidance[13] states that "all general hospitals need to have isolation facilities available either in suitable side rooms on general wards, in separate isolation wards or both." Health and Safety at Work legislation requires hospital management to ensure that formal risk assessments are carried out and arrangements are in place to minimise the risk of transmission of infection to patients and staff. The nature and extent of isolation facilities available needs to be considered as part of this assessment.[1]

Patients may be nursed in isolation if they have a disease or condition that has the potential to spread or because they are highly susceptible to acquiring an infection as a result of their underlying condition or therapy. Isolation of patients may be required on admission of a patient with a particular infection in order to prevent the spread to other in-patients, and for those patients who develop an infection during their hospital stay.[1]

The House of Lords Select Committee report[21] stated that "Isolation of patients is an expensive but effective form of infection control." However, there is a lack of evidence based research on how best and when to use isolation facilities cost effectively. The National Audit Office found that isolation facilities in some NHS Trusts have been significantly reduced over the last five to six years. Some infection control teams believe this lack of facilities has created a serious problem, especially in their efforts to deal with MRSA. They also found little evaluation of the cost-effectiveness of closing isolation facilities.[1] Furthermore, because of bed shortages,[22] isolation rooms may be used for other patients. Speaking at the conference Dr Louise Teare, Consultant Microbiologist at the Mid-Essex Trust suggested the need to introduce MRSA free zones on surgical wards. She illustrated how she is working with clinical teams in her Trust and has started to separate out elective and emergency patients on orthopaedic wards in order to help reduce infection rates. They are also introducing visitor restrictions and a particular type of uniform for staff. The aim is to change the culture of these teams.

In response to the Committee of Public Accounts questioning, the Department acknowledged that where there was greater opportunity to isolate people in smaller rooms or single rooms, hospitals could avoid the spread of infection by getting the physical layout of the room right.[7] They noted that this will in future be facilitated as part of the current system of planning of health services as the current trend is for smaller patient rooms with en-suite facilities. They also pointed out that there had already been an investment in isolation facilities in specialist children's hospitals but they accepted that if there was to be more investment in infection control then part should be in isolation facilities.[7] The Department's Action plan, HSC 2000/002,[9] included as one of its objectives the need to secure appropriate provision of isolation facilities within each Trust. This required Chief Executives, working with infection control teams, to undertake risk assessments to determine appropriate provision and agree the level and type of provision with Regional Offices by 1 June 2000.

Screening can be an important tool in helping to reduce hospital acquired infection

Screening involves taking swabs from asymptomatic patients and staff that are then subjected to microbiological testing to determine whether they are colonised or infected by specific micro-organisms. While patients can be screened for any infection, the main focus of regular screening by Trusts was for MRSA.[4] Some infection control teams told the National Audit Office that they saw screening patients as an infection control measure that had been successful in reducing MRSA infection rates in their NHS Trust. For example, Kings' College Hospital considers screening to be a cost effective measure in reducing infection rates and has set up a process dedicated to screening for MRSA, with some 15,000 tests carried out each year costing about £120,000 per annum. Other NHS Trusts have used screening in a cost effective way in high-risk situations.[1]

Screening patients, however, can prove expensive and a number of infection control teams questioned whether it was always of value, believing that actively screening patients, other than in high-risk situations, had no impact on their infection rates. While there is guidance on screening in high-risk situations, there is no guidance about screening in general and a need for evidence based research to inform screening policies to determine when it is likely to be cost effective.[1]

Summary and conclusions

While not all hospital acquired infection can be prevented this chapter illustrates how better information and knowledge about realistic infection control practices can improve prevention. This in turn should lead to improved patient outcomes and release resources which can subsequently be used to treat other patients. The prevention and control of hospital acquired infection take many different forms and operates at different levels in the health care system. For example, improving environmental cleanliness is an issue which needs to be addressed through the management of the cleaning contracts whereas hand hygiene, which is possibly one of the most important interventions, is something that all staff should comply with.

Evidence of non-compliance with these and other strategies, and poor understanding of the problem, suggest that education needs to be improved. This in turn would assist in raising the profile of hospital acquired infection and potentially, lead to improvements in prevention and control. Of particular importance here is the need for a concerted effort to tackle the rise of antibiotic resistant micro-organisms through the prudent use of antibiotics, infection control and surveillance.

Key points:

■ all Trusts should consider whether their employees ought to have compliance with good infection control and prevention practices included as part of their job descriptions;

■ infection control teams need to provide, and all Trust employees need to access, education and training on hospital acquired infection, including ensuring compliance with HSC 2000/002;

■ NHS Trusts need to ensure that written information on infection control policies and procedures are available to all staff;

■ Trusts need to ensure compliance with the NHS Plan Implementation targets aimed at improving hospital cleanliness. infection control teams will need to input into audits aimed at monitoring compliance with the Trust Cleanliness Action Plan and ensure that the results are fed back to the Trust Board and communicated to all staff;

■ infection control teams need to liaise with hospital pharmacies to ensure that audits of antibiotic prescribing and monitoring of links with antibiotic resistance are undertaken and continue to implement action set out in HSC 1999/049 and HSC 2000/002;

■ Trusts need to review the adequacy of their isolation facilities, undertaking risk assessments as specified in HSC 2000/002; and

■ Trusts need to review the effectiveness of their screening policies.

Chapter 6
Maintaining the initiative

Hospital acquired infections are a serious issue

The best available data suggest that at any one time nine per cent of patients have a hospital acquired infection.[1] There are at least 300,000 hospital acquired infections each year,[7] and an estimated 5,000 patients die each year as a direct result of acquiring an infection during their hospital stay.[13] The cost to the NHS of dealing with the effects of hospital acquired infection is at least £1 billion. While there will always be an irreducible minimum level of infection, the National Audit Office estimated that a 15 per cent reduction is possible.[1] These data, together with the fact that hospital acquired infections can have a significant impact on the Trust's other policies, highlight that this is a very significant issue with serious implications for patients and for the NHS.

Putting hospital acquired infection on the NHS agenda

Hospital acquired infection is now firmly on the NHS agenda. The Department's Action Plan for the NHS, published in February 2000, set out a programme of action aimed at improving each Trust's approach to the management and control of hospital acquired infection.[9] A core requirement in the December 2000 NHS Plan Implementation Programme[6] is the need for all relevant organisations to ensure that they have effective systems in place, including decontamination, to prevent and control communicable diseases, especially hospital acquired infection, so as to minimise the risk of infection to patients and others. Organisations also need to take action to control and reduce antimicrobial resistance and meet immunisation targets.

Initiatives that aim to ensure improved management and control of hospital acquired infection

The House of Lords Select Committee on Science and Technology report on their 1998 Inquiry into Resistance to Antibiotics and other Antimicrobial Agents[21] and the Government's response[52] were significant events in raising the profile of hospital acquired infection. Since then, the Department has issued information and guidance to NHS Trusts and commissioners of health care, culminating in the introduction of Clinical Governance,[11] the Controls Assurance Standards[12] and the Department's Action plan HSC 2000/002.[9] These emphasise the actions that need to be taken if the management and control of hospital acquired infection is to improve, and in the case of the HSC 2000/002, specifies particular targets. The National Audit Office report[1] and Committee of Public Accounts hearing and report[7] were important milestones in highlighting the lack of grip on the extent and cost of the problem and the issues that need to be addressed at NHS Trust level.

Compliance at NHS Trust level varies

Evidence presented in the National Audit Office report[1] and at the conference indicated that at Trust level hospital acquired infection is still afforded a low status. There remains a general lack of awareness of the scale of the problem and the socio-economic burden imposed. The National Audit Office report acknowledged the dedication of infection control nurses and doctors in preventing and minimising the problem of hospital acquired infection. However, they concluded that infection control did not appear to have the attention it warrants, that there appeared to be a mismatch between what was expected of infection control teams and the resources allocated to them, and there seemed to be difficulties in translating policies into effective practice.

Adequate resources are needed

A recurrent theme throughout the National Audit Office conference, was that the levels of resources allocated to infection control were insufficient to enable infection control teams to fulfil their responsibilities, including surveillance, the provision of education and training and prevention activities. The NHS has been promised more resources and John Denham MP, the then Health Minister, suggested that some of these resources should be directed specifically towards infection control. While resourcing should be linked to identified needs, targeted investment in infection control is likely to reap substantial benefits both in terms of improved patient outcomes and the release of resources for alternative use. Benefits should also be felt from resources that are ploughed into other areas within individual Trusts, for example, the "Clean Hospitals" initiative. Graham Elderfield Chief Executive of the Isle of Wight Healthcare NHS Trust, suggested that it was inappropriate to ask whether we can afford investment in infection control, arguing that we can't afford to dis-invest in this area.

There is a need for robust comparable data and adoption of appropriate surveillance

The Department's 1995 guidance[13] and subsequent circulars, such as HSC 2000/002,[9] have stressed the importance of surveillance of infection. The National Audit Office[1] described surveillance as key to an effective infection control programme and many speakers referred to the importance of this activity and, in particular, the benefits of a national surveillance scheme that enables valid comparisons of infection rates at different hospitals to be made. The information generated should be used to inform infection control programmes. In particular, hospitals with higher than average infection rates should use this information as a trigger to investigate why this should be the case and subsequently implement a programme of intervention to address the problem.

The Nosocomial Infection National Surveillance Scheme for NHS Hospitals in England was set up in November 1995 and the first surveillance module launched in May 1997. Since its launch 179 NHS Trusts have participated in one or more modules. The Committee of Public Accounts welcomed the introduction of a national scheme and recommended that participation should be made mandatory,[7] a sentiment endorsed by John Denham MP.[33] The Committee of Public Accounts were told that the scheme is now entering a new phase, one that it is hoped will evolve into a truly national service.[8] This should facilitate surveillance at the local level and through this process generate regional and national surveillance databases, against which individual Trusts can assess their own performance, and a national picture can be developed and monitored. The new compulsory service was launched on 1 April 2001, with the first national data on bacteraemia infections expected in April 2002.

If it is to be effective, the overall aim of this service needs to made clear. It needs to improve patient care by assisting hospitals to change clinical practice, and as such reduce the risk of acquiring a hospital infection and consequencly reduce rates, by providing national statistics on hospital acquired infection for comparison with local results. It is also important that the Department identifies and makes explicit the objectives of any new surveillance scheme, and that Trusts understand how the data are to be used and what resources will need to be deployed in collecting the data.

chapter six

There is a need for everyone to accept responsibility for implementing effective infection control arrangements

The failure of healthcare workers to recognise that the prevention and control of hospital acquired infection is everybody's responsibility and not just that of infection control teams was seen to be an important obstacle to improving infection control. Of particular concern was the lack of involvement of the Chief Executive in infection control issues in some NHS Trusts.[1]

The Department's 1995 guidance recommended that the Trust Chief Executive or a nominated deputy should be a member of the Hospital Infection Control Committee and that Chief Executives should approve the annual infection control programme.[13] The National Audit Office found that this was often not the case.[1] Speakers at the conference emphasised the need for Chief Executives of all NHS Trusts to take an active role in the management and control of hospital acquired infection. The Department told the Committee of Public Accounts, and reiterated the message at the conference, that the adoption of clinical governance and controls assurance initiatives should ensure greater compliance by making the Chief Executive explicitly responsible for infection control.[8]

Initiatives aimed at tackling antibiotic resistance need to be rigorously pursued

The House of Lords Select Committee on Science and Technology highlighted concerns about the global rise of antibiotic resistance.[21] These concerns were also raised in the National Audit Office report[1] and Committee of Public Accounts hearing.[8] A number of speakers at the National Audit Office conference provided examples of why these concerns need to be acted upon. For example, antibiotic resistance:

■ makes infections more difficult to treat;

■ may prolong or prohibit recovery, and increase the period of infectiousness, putting others at increased risk of infection;

■ places the individual at increased risk of complications, either as a direct result of the treatment they receive and/or their prolonged recovery period; and

■ in some cases may result in a prolonged in-patient stay and higher treatment costs, thereby placing an additional burden on scarce health resources.

The UK Strategy for tackling antimicrobial resistance[2] involves a three pronged approach: surveillance of infection; effective infection control; and the prudent use of antibiotics facilitated by antibiotic policies and other factors, including education of the public into issues relating to appropriate antibiotics use and the danger of inappropriate use. Launched at the National Audit Office conference, the UK Strategy has received unanimous support and agreement.

There is a need for adequate education and training of all staff

The poor knowledge of clinical staff about the control of infection and their non-compliance with effective infection control activities has been identified as another impediment to achieving good infection control. The need for greater compliance has been clearly evidenced and a key way is to ensure that all health care workers receive appropriate education and training, including appropriate education and training during their induction period and annual update sessions. The National Audit Office found that whilst infection control nurses recognised the importance of providing such sessions, a considerable proportion of NHS Trusts failed to provide adequate levels of education to staff within their Trust.[1] While the use of interactive computer technology may further assist in this process there is a need to facilitate appropriate access to-up-to-date information on the nature of the problem and for guidance to be available 24 hours a day.

Other factors that may facilitate increased awareness of hospital acquired infection issues include improving undergraduate education and training. Susan Macqueen, the then Chair of the Infection Control Nurses Association, explained how they were trying to ensure that increased emphasis was given to infection control issues within undergraduate nurse training.

There is a need to be aware of the conflicts between policies

The prospect that policies directed towards achieving the Trust's other targets may conflict with those directed towards promoting a reduction in infection, needs to be addressed.[1] For example, tackling waiting lists was identified as a 'must do' in the NHS Plan Implementation Programme[6] document. However, achieving a reduction in waiting lists may result in a faster turnover of patients, the more intensive use of beds, and the transfer of patients between wards, resulting in an increased intensity of workload and possibly an increase in the risk of infection.

Specific activities that work

The audit of infection prevention and control activities can provide valuable information that can be used to assess progress and indicate areas for action. The adoption of surveillance and participation in the national surveillance scheme will contribute to this process by quantifying the effects of these activities and enabling infection rates to be calculated to determine the level of improvements made. Comparisons with a benchmark derived from the accumulated rates from other hospitals will indicate whether further interventions are necessary.

Other aspects of infection control also need to be monitored. In particular, there is a need to examine the management framework again and assess whether it is working. Within NHS Trusts there is perhaps a need to audit and assess the standing of infection control and whether it has improved. Key questions are:

- is hospital acquired infection getting the attention it deserves?

- are Chief Executives actively involved in these issues?

- are hospital acquired infection issues discussed regularly at Board level?

- is the Hospital Infection Control Committee functioning effectively?

- are infection control teams adequately resourced?

- are infection control teams able to fulfil their remit and, in particular, have they been able to increase their commitment to proactive infection control activities rather than spend the vast majority of their time engaged in reacting to situations?

- has staff awareness and understanding of the problem of hospital acquired infection increased?

- what is the level of compliance with effective infection control activities?

The Committee of Public Accounts recognised that a number of initiatives were being adopted and that the impact of these may not be seen until 2003 but they considered that progress was essential if the NHS was to meet its duty and commitment to patients. They expect a report on progress by 2003.[7]

Responsibility for monitoring the implementation of the controls assurance standard on infection control through the NHS performance management process, rests with the Commission for Health Improvement and the Audit Commission.[12] The Department expects this monitoring to provide valuable data on infection prevention and control arrangements and how these change over time. The information generated may then be used to inform future guidance.

Concluding remarks

The evidence clearly demonstrates that hospital acquired infections are a substantial drain on healthcare resources and place a financial and non-financial burden on patients and their carers. It is equally evident that, while not all hospital acquired infections are avoidable, a proportion can be prevented through effective infection prevention and control activities. Although there are inevitably costs associated with achieving a reduction in hospital acquired infection rates, the net benefits are likely to remain significantly large.

Hospital acquired infection is now firmly on the NHS agenda. The task now is to raise the status of hospital acquired infection at Trust level, to increase awareness of hospital acquired infection issues, and to foster a culture where all health care workers appreciate that they have a responsibility for the prevention and control of hospital acquired infection. An appropriate management framework and an appropriately resourced and informed infection control programme that crosses budgetary and professional boundaries should help facilitate this process.

Intrinsic and extrinsic risk factors for infections are constantly changing and a dynamic approach to the prevention and control of hospital acquired infection is required. A programme of evaluation at Trust and national level should provide important data on progress, inform future action and enhance the ability to prevent and control these infections and ultimately improve patient care. The Committee of Public Accounts raised a number of issues,[7] which the Department plan to respond to by providing a number of reports updating them on various situations.[8] This will continue to keep the issues in the audit arena. The information contained in this book is intended to help maintain the momentum and ensure that the challenge of hospital acquired infection continues to be met.

Managing and controlling

HOSPITAL ACQUIRED INFECTION

The way ahead

ADDITION TO ADVERTISED PROGRAMME

John Denham MP, Minister of State for Health, will be speaking to the conference about the importance which the Government attaches to the task of tackling hospital acquired infection, and their new strategy to address the problem of antimicrobial resistance.

The Minister will speak at 16.40

This will be followed by a summary of the day's events by
Dr James Robertson, NAO.
Delegates are then invited to attend an informal reception at
the conference centre from 17.15 - 18.30

Monday 12 June 2000

The QEII Conference Centre, London

CME
Accredita
applied
for

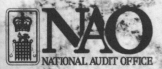

NATIONAL AUDIT OFFICE

This conference is based on the findings of *The Management and Control of Hospital Acquired Infection in Acute NHS Trusts in England* report published by the National Audit Office on 14 February 2000.

Appendix 1

The conference programme

The management and control of hospital acquired infection: The Way Ahead

Monday, 12 June 2000
QE II Conference Centre, London

9.30   **Welcome and Opening Remarks**
Sir John Bourn, Comptroller and Auditor General National Audit Office

9.40   **Key recommendations from the NAO report, and the Committee of Public Accounts hearing on the Management & Control of Hospital Acquired Infection**
Karen Taylor, Audit Manager Health VFM Audit National Audit Office

■ what do we need to know about hospital acquired infection?

■ what are the constraints to applying existing guidelines, standards & arrangements?

■ what solutions did the report identify?

10.00   **Controlling hospital acquired infection: the Department of Health's strategy**
Dr Pat Troop, Deputy Chief Medical Officer The Department of Health

■ strengthening arrangements for the prevention and control of infection in hospitals

■ improving surveillance of hospital infection

Questions & Answers

10.30   The strategic management of hospital acquired infection
Four, fifteen minute presentations

Chairman **Dr Pat Troop,** Deputy Chief Medical Officer The Department of Health

Controls assurance and eliminating the risk of hospital acquired infection
Stuart Emslie, Head of Controls Assurance NHS Executive

What do the NAO report, and the controls assurance standards, mean for Chief Executives?
Graham Elderfield, Chief Executive Isle of Wight Healthcare NHS Trust

Advice for Chief Executives & clinicians: how to progress the hospital acquired infection agenda
Professor Gary French, Chairman Hospital Infection Society

The role of nurses: how should they respond to the hospital acquired infection agenda?
Susan Macqueen, Clinical Nurse Specialist - Infection Control, Great Ormond Street Hospital for Children NHS Trust, and Chair The Infection Control Nurses Association

Questions & Answers

12.30   **Lunch**

13.30   The importance of surveillance in helping to reduce hospital acquired infection
Four, fifteen minute presentations

Chairman **Dr Lindsey Davies,** Regional Director of Public Health The Department of Health

Developing national surveillance of hospital acquired infection
Professor Brian Duerden, Deputy Director Public Health
Laboratory Service

**The implications of the current results of the Nosocomial
Infection National Surveillance Scheme**
Dr Andrew Pearson, Head Nosocomial Infection National
Surveillance Unit, Public Health Laboratory Service

Surveillance and feedback to clinicians: the question of ownership
Dr Edward T M Smyth, Consultant Bacteriologist & Infection
Control Doctor The Royal Hospitals Trust, Belfast

Engaging clinicians: the views of an infection control nurse
Jennifer Wilson, Senior Nurse Manager & Surveillance Co-
ordinator Nosocomial Infection Surveillance Unit

Questions & Answers

Key messages to take away
Three, fifteen minute presentations

Chairman **Lord Soulsby of Swaffam Prior,** President The Royal
Society of Medicine and Chairman The House of Lords Select
Committee on Science & Technology Inquiry (1988) into Resistance
to Antibiotics & other Antimicrobial Agents

15.30   **Are the bugs winning?**
         Lord Soulsby of Swaffam Prior

15.45   **The impact of restrictive antibiotic policies on infection control**
         Dr Geoff Scott, Consultant Microbiologist University College
         London Hospitals NHS Trust

How to raise the profile of infection control and improve patient care
Dr Louise Teare, Consultant Microbiologist Mid-Essex Hospitals NHS Trust

16.40   **The importance which the Government attaches to the task of tackling hospital acquired infection and their new strategy to address the problem of antimicrobial resistance**

John Denham MP, Minister of State for Health

Questions & Answers

17.00   **What next: the summary of the day's events**

James Robertson, Director Health VFM National Audit Office

Appendix 2

Comparison of the Committee of Public Accounts report recommendations on the management and control of hospital acquired infection and the Government's Treasury Minute response

Committee of Public Accounts Report Recommendations[7]

> i Research indicates that between 50 per cent and 70 per cent of surgical wound infections occur post-discharge, but these infections are not monitored. The NHS Executive are undertaking research into post-discharge infection, and we look forward to seeing the outcome later this year. We recommend that post-discharge infections are monitored in future through the national surveillance scheme.

Government's Treasury Minute Response[8]

The Department funded report referred to by the Committee has just been received by the Department and is currently being subject to peer review. A copy of the final report will be sent to the Committee as soon as it is finalised. It is well recognised in published literature that once a patient has left the confines of a hospital it is difficult to ensure accuracy in surveillance of any post-discharge infection. However, a UK-wide meeting of consultant microbiologists and others with a key interest in this area was held in Glasgow on 16 January 2001 to review progress and make recommendations. The NHS Healthcare Associated Surveillance Group referred to below will now take this work forward.

Committee of Public Accounts Report Recommendations[7]

ii The NHS Executive have now taken action to improve surveillance, including researching the links between antimicrobial resistance and prescribing, measuring infections that occur after patients have been discharged from hospital, and doubling their investment in the Nosocomial Infection National Surveillance Scheme. But by December 1999, only 139 self-selecting Acute NHS Trusts in England were participating in the surveillance scheme. We recognise that the Executive are expanding the Scheme, but we believe that they should go further and make it mandatory.

Government's Treasury Minute Response[8]

The Minister of State for Health announced in September that surveillance of hospital acquired infection would be made compulsory for all NHS Acute Trusts from 1 April 2001 and that data would be published from 1 April 2002. A new NHS Healthcare Associated Infection Surveillance Steering Group, chaired by an NHS Chief Executive, was set up in September 2000 to provide the Department with urgent recommendations on infection surveillance needs at local, regional and national level, building on improving on the limited coverage of the current Nosocomial Infection National Surveillance Scheme, to deliver national surveillance reporting of hospital acquired infection by all Acute Trusts from 1 April 2001. Details of the proposed arrangements will be announced shortly.

Committee of Public Accounts Report Recommendations[7]

iii The NHS Executive acknowledge that it should be possible to reduce the incidence of hospital acquired infection by 15 per or more, avoiding costs of some £150 million and saving lives. Since 1996, and particularly since 1998, the NHS Executive have taken a series of actions and initiatives to address this issue, but do not expect to see tangible, measurable progress until 2003. Such progress will be essential for the NHS to meet their duty and commitment to patients.

Government's Treasury Minute Response[8]

In his report in February 2000, the C&AG estimated that 15 per cent of hospital acquired infection could be prevented. This was based on a bed weighted average of responses from 174 Infection Control Teams in Acute NHS Trusts. The report suggests that potential avoidable costs are around £150 million a year. However, this figure should be treated with caution because it was derived from research on the socio-economic burden of hospital acquired infection at one hospital - and subsequently extrapolated across the rest of the NHS where costs vary widely from hospital to hospital.

The Department nevertheless accepts that the incidence of hospital acquired infection can be reduced significantly with associated cost savings and, indeed, as the Committee acknowledge, a wide range of action is already in hand to this end. The subject is, as the Committee say, now firmly in focus. The recently published Implementation Programme for the NHS Plan makes it very clear that, as one of the core requirements underpinning the NHS targets set out in the NHS Plan, all relevant organisations must have effective systems in place to prevent and control hospital acquired infection. At local level, this is the responsibility of each Trust and its Chief Executive. The Department is considering how best to strengthen current NHS performance management arrangements for infection control. Details of the arrangements in place at each Trust will be available to the Commission for Health Improvement as part of its clinical governance review processes and to the Audit Commission in their reviews of provider care.

Tangible, measurable progress in tackling Hospital Acquired Infection is already being delivered. For example, in response to the NHS action plans: Resistance to Antibiotics and other Antimicrobial Agents and; Management and Control of Hospital Acquired Infection (Health Service Circulars 1999/049 and 2000/002 respectively), there has been good progress in a number of areas, including:

■ an increase in NHS Trust Chief Executive/senior management commitment to infection control, eg. 63 per cent attending Infection Control Committee meetings at the time of the Comptroller and Auditor General's study, is now reported as 91 per cent;

■ NHS Trusts are actively putting in place Infection Control Programmes for 2001-02, including measures to redress any shortfalls in meeting the relevant Control Assurances Infection Control Standard;

■ an increase in IT, clerical and secretarial support to Infection Control Teams;

- Infection Control Teams are now being consulted more frequently by senior management on service development issues eg. on the purchase of equipment for clinical areas;

- the need for isolation facilities is being addressed;

- most NHS Trusts have in the last two years undertaken initiatives or programmes on handwashing.

The Department will continue to closely monitor progress to ensure that robust and effective infection control arrangements are in place across the country to protect the health of patients, staff and visitors.

Committee of Public Accounts Report Recommendations[7]

> iv Key to achieving progress will be the effective implementation of the new Controls Assurance System, which builds on the statutory duty of chief executives for quality of care. This will raise the profile of hospital acquired infection, especially in the 20 per cent of Acute NHS Trusts tha do not have a strategy for dealing with it. Every Trust has to have a plan in place by July 2000 setting out priorities for action and produce an annual report on progress, priorities and key issues by the end of April 2003.

Government's Treasury Minute Response[8]

As part of the controls assurance process for 1999-2000, NHS organisations were required to self-assess against a number of standards, including one on infecton control and, for identified deficiencies, produce a prioritised action plan with timescales and clearly defined responsibilities.

The datahas been analysed centrally and Regional Offices are now following up identified deficiencies with the Trust concerned as part of the NHS performance review process. Progress will be reported to the Committee as requested.

The NHS Litigation Authority (NHSLA), which has issued a number of standards for assessing the effectiveness of risk management insupport of the Clinical Negligence Scheme for Trusts (CNST), has recently revised these standards drawing on key aspects of the Department's Controls Assurance Infection Control Standard and Health Service Circular 2000/02 (see paragraph 69). The NHSLA will begin to assess Trust against these revised standards during the 2001-02 financial year.

Committee of Public Accounts Recommendations[7]

> v   Complacency, poor prescribing practice and misuse of antibiotics has led to the emergence of drug resistant infections. As the Chief Medical Officer told us, there are no simple solutions any more. The NHS Executive have now launched initiatives to look at the more prudent use of antibiotics, and to monitor and control prescribing including the new Government strategy to tackle antibiotic resistant infections announced in June 2000. We expect this work to lead to evidence-based guidance on effective prescribing strategies.

Government's Treasury Minute Response[8]

The UK Antimicrobial Resistance Strategy and Action Plan published in June 2000, to which the Committee refers, outlined the areas where work is underway to promote optimal antimicrobial prescribing in clinical practice. An Interdepartmental Steering Group (IDSG) is overseeing and co-ordinating work on the Strategy.

Twelve months ago the IDSG set up a Clinical Prescribing Group which is looking at ways of optimising and monitoring prescribing of antimicrobials in clinical practice through professional education, promotion of evidence-based guidelines, prescribing and organisational support and surveillance. As part of this, the Public Health Laboratory Service (PHLS) has developed and distributed a template intended to be used as a basis for the development of local evidence-based antimicrobial prescribing policies in primary care. It is available on the PHLS website and will be reviewed in the light of comments received and updated as the evidence-base evolves. PHLS has also organised a series of workshops with local healthcare professionals on the use of antibiotics in primary care.

The National Prescribing Centre (NPC) has developed a tool kit providing clinical audit guidance on antimicrobial prescribing and monitoring. This has been disseminated to all Health Authorities (HAs), Primary Care Groups/Trusts (PCGs/Ts) and hospital trusts. A change management resource pack has also been developed by the NPC, in which the prudent prescribing of antimicrobial agents is used as an illustrative example. The NPC has run four full-day therapeutics seminars for HA and senior PCG/T prescribing advisors this year on the proper use of antimicrobials. Nineteen senior prescribing advisors have been recruited by the NPC and given two days intensive training plus materials; they will each present at and lead a minimum of two half-day seminars for PCG prescribing advisors and practice-based pharmacists on the appropriate use of antimicrobials and use of the audit materials.

appendices

Committee of Public Accounts Report Recommendations[7]

> vi Hospital hygiene is crucial in preventing hospital acquired infection, including basic practice such as handwashing. We find it inexcusable that compliance with guidance on handwashing is so poor. We note the steps the Executive have now taken to improve awareness and education, but look to them to audit progress and report back to us by the end of 2001.

Government's Treasury Minute Response[8]

The Controls Assurance Standard on Infection Control expects Trusts to have a policy on hand hygiene, and to provide education and training in this area and on the prevention and control of infection generally to all staff. Compliance will be monitored by internal audit and the new NHS performance management process. As stated in paragraph 4, the arrangements are also open to review by the Commission for Health Improvement and the Audit Commission. Progress will be reported to the Committee as requested.

New evidence based guidelines for the prevention and control of hospital acquired infection were published as a supplement to the Journal of Hospital Infection in January 2001. The guidelines include the standard principles of infection control, including hand hygiene.

The guidelines have been distributed with a joint letter from the Chief Medical Officer and Chief Nursing Office to a range of health care professionals, including Infection Control Nurses, Infection Control Doctors and Clinical Governance leads. The guidelines can also be used as an audit toll of clinical practice and be incorporated into local clinical governance programmes. The guidelines will be reviewed in two years time as part of the National Institute of Clinical Excellences (NICE) work programme.

A summary of the guidelines will also be published in the Nursing Times early in 2001. A Department commissioned poster on the "Top Ten" most important infection control interventions, including hand hygiene, is being prepared and will be distributed with every edition of the Nursing Times. One of the aims of this initiative will be to have a copy of the poster on every hospital ward across the NHS.

£31 million was allocated directly to NHS Trusts in July 2000 to secure improvements in the patient's environment including levels of hygiene and cleanliness. A further £30 million is being allocated next year to ensure that these targets are met.

Committee of Public Accounts Report Recommendations[7]

> vii The increased priority and attention that is rightly now being given to hospital acquired infection has not been matched by resources. Some new money, £5 million over two years, has been allocated, some extra infection control nurses have been appointed, and the Executive accept the case for investment in smaller wards and isolation facilities. The scale of hospital acquired infection calls for sufficient funding to ensure that hospitals can tackle the problem effectively, and so reduce the impact on patients and NHS costs.

Government's Treasury Minute Response[8]

The Department welcomes the Committee's acknowledgement of the high priority which it is now giving to combating hospital acquired infection, and agrees that this needs to be matched by appropriate funding locally. Over the next four years the service will receive its largest ever level of sustained real-terms growth, averaging six point three per cent year on year - a step change in the resources available for the NHS. It is not possible for the Department to make sensible judgements about how much of this needs to be spent at each hospital in order to achieve targets they have been set. However, the Department expect the Chief Executive of each NHS Trust to spend what is necessary to do that, and has charged each one individually to deliver. The £5 million, which is being used mainly to fund development initiatives, therefore represents only a very small proportion of the total additional resources which will be spent to ensure that effective systems are in place to prevent and control hospital acquired infection. An additional £1 million has been allocated through the Department's Regional Offices to secure improvements in infection control training.

Committee of Public Accounts Report Recommendations[7]

> viii The NHS Executive recognise that more effective bed management can help reduce hospital acquired infection. Greater use of smaller rooms and single bed rooms is now part of health service planning, and the Executive accept that increased investment in isolation facilities is a priority. But high throughput of patients is also a factor. As we noted in our report on Inpatient Admissions, Bed Management and Patient Discharge, some hospitals are operating at very high levels of bed occupancy. Wider application of best practice will help Acute Trusts manage beds better. Trusts also need to ensure that infection control is an integral part of their bed management policies.

Government's Treasury Minute Response[8]

Through the National Booked Admissions Programme, NHS Trusts are taking forward work on the relationship between demand and supply in order to schedule work more effectively. Central to this is effective bed management. Best practice will be shared through the Modernisation Agency.

Current bed occupancy in general and acute beds is around 83.1 per cent (1999-2000). However, the NHS Plan provision for an additional 2,100 general and acute beds by 2003-04 will enable, among other things, the occupancy rate to be reduced to 82 per cent, significantly improving bed availability in hospitals and the management of emergency and elective workloads. National Beds Inquiry planning guidance to be issued soon will help Health Authorities to consider where extra beds are required. NHS Estates is currently developing guidance on ways in which the built environment can assist with the control of infection.

Committee of Public Accounts Report Recommendations[7]

> ix   The Chief Medical Officer accepts that in staffing infection control teams, a ratio of one nurse to 250 beds is a good benchmark for NHS Trusts. But many Trusts have much larger numbers of beds per nurse. While local variations in circumstances and practice may account for some of these variations, we expect the NHS Executive to carry out further research, in conjunction with the Infection Control Nurses Association, with the aim of developing staffing guidelines for Trusts.

Government's Treasury Minute Response[8]

It is for NHS Trusts and Health Authorities, who are accountable for the quality of services they provide, to decide on the number, grade and mix of staff they require, to provide this service to patients.

The Department will have discussions with the Infection Control Nurses Association and other professional organisations about the development of an assessment tool for NHS Trusts to help them to reach decisions about staffing levels and skill mix required within their Infection Control Teams.

Appendix 3

Department of Health initiatives: 1988 - December 1999

- In 1988, a Joint Working Group set up by the then Department of Health and Social Security and the Public Health Laboratory Service produced the first national guidance on infection control in hospitals, including the need to establish Infection Control Committees and infection control teams.

- In 1993, an Infection Control Standards Working Group comprising the Association of Medical Microbiologists, Hospital Infection Society, Infection Control Nurses Association and Public Health Laboratory Service, issued "Standards in Infection Control in Hospitals." While not issued by the Department of Health, the standards were acknowledged by them as providing a suitable framework for infection control teams to follow.

- In March 1995, the Hospital Infection Working Group of the Department and Public Health Laboratory Service issued revised Hospital Infection Control Guidance. The guidance, known as the Cooke Report, was issued under cover of HSG(95) 10 with the statement that this was "now Department of Health policy on infection control." This guidance strengthened the 1988 guidance and included new advice on improving surveillance of hospital acquired infection.

- In March 1996, the Department of Health and Public Health Laboratory Service established the Nosocomial Infection National Surveillance Scheme to improve patient care by helping hospitals to reduce rates and risk of hospital acquired infection. This was the first attempt to produce national data on hospital acquired infection for comparison with local results. The first Annual Reports on bacteraemia and surgical site infections were published in May and December 1999.

- In 1997, the Department commissioned regional epidemiologists to examine communicable disease control services provided by local health authorities throughout England. The survey identified a number of shortcomings and that communicable disease control was hard pressed in some areas. The results of this study have been considered by Regional Offices and action is being taken to address identified shortcomings.

- In 1997 and 1998, the Government's NHS Priorities and Planning Guidance made it clear that health authorities must satisfy themselves that appropriate arrangements are in place for communicable disease control. In particular, the "National Priorities Guidance for 1999/00-2001/02" (HSC(98)159: LAC(98)22), issued in September 1998, required health authorities to ensure "continuing and effective protection of the public health with particular regard to the prevention and control of hospital infection, communicable diseases, antibiotic resistance and the effects of environmental and chemical hazards."

- In February 1998, the Department commissioned the production of evidence-based guidelines on the general principles for preventing hospital-acquired infections. The guidelines which contain many elements of clinical practice for preventing the spread of hospital-acquired infection, including multi-drug resistant organisms, were expected to be completed in summer 2000. The project has been extended and guidelines have been commissioned for the prevention and control of infection in primary and community care settings.

- In June 1998, the Department commissioned regional epidemiologists to examine infection control arrangements in NHS Trusts. The results of this study have been considered by Regional Directors of Public Health and an action plan is being taken forward to address areas where shortcomings were identified.

- In September 1998, following a request from the then Chief Medical Officer, the Standing Medical Advisory Committee (SMAC) produced its report "The Path of Least Resistance." The report examined antimicrobial resistance in relation to medical prescribing. The report stressed that effective infection control was fundamental to preventing the spread of resistant organisms.

- In December 1998, the House of Lords Select Committee on Science and Technology published a report on their Inquiry into "Resistance to Antibiotics and other Antimicrobial agents", in response the Government re-affirmed that infection control and hygiene should be a core management responsibility.

- In 1998, health protection arrangements were considered as part of the Chief Medical Officer's project to strengthen the public health function. One of the main recommendations was the development of a communicable disease strategy and work on this is in progress.

- In March 1999, the Department issued HSC 1999/049 detailing action for the NHS following the Government's response to the House of Lords report and the SMAC report, "The Path of Least Resistance." Regional Offices are in the process of implementing action plans.

■ In May 1999, as part of Governance in the new NHS, the Department issued HSC 1999/123 setting out action for NHS Trusts and health authorities for 1999-2000 in respect of moving beyond financial controls assurance statements to the production of statements covering wider organisational controls, including risk management.

■ In November 1999, the Department issued further guidance, supplementing HSC 1999/123. New risk management and organisational standards, including controls assurance standards for infection control, were launched and sent out to the NHS.

■ In December 1999, the Government published "Modernising Health and Social Services: National Priorities Guidance 2000-01 and 2002-03". This stressed the importance of working in partnership to "strengthen services to prevent and control communicable diseases, especially hospital acquired infection, taking action to reduce antimicrobial resistance..." (HSC(99)242:LAC(99)38).

This Table appeared originally in the National Audit Office report.[1]

Glossary

Acute beds
Includes beds on the following wards: Intensive Care, terminally ill/palliative care, all acute surgical and medical and paediatric, acute maternity and acute elderly and young physically disabled.

Acute NHS Trust
Hospitals which are managed by their own Boards and which provide acute beds linked to medical and surgical intervention.

Acquired antibiotic resistance
Resistance to anti microbial agents that develops in micro-organisms that were previously sensitive.

Agency nurse
Temporary nursing staff booked by the NHS Trust from a commercial employment agency to provide holiday cover or to deal with temporary staff shortages.

Alert condition surveillance
Specific infections or other illnesses which the hospital ward staff are required to report to the infection control team.

Alert organism surveillance
Specific organisms which microbiology laboratory staff are required to report to the infection control team.

Antibiotic
A substance that selectively destroys or inhibits the growth of certain bacteria.

Antibiotic policy
Written guidance that recommends antibiotics and their dosage for treating and preventing specific infections.

Antimicrobial agent Any compound that selectively destroys or inhibits the growth of micro-organisms.

Audit Organised review of current practices and comparisons with pre-determined standards. Action is then taken to rectify any deficiencies that have been identified in current practices. The review is repeated to see if the pre-determined standards are being met.

Audit Commission A statutory body whose functions include oversight of the external audit of NHS Trusts and health authorities in England and Wales. In addition it carries out value for money studies in different aspects of health and local government services.

Bacteraemia Presence of bacteria in the bloodstream.

Bacterium (Bacteria) A simple microscopic single-celled organism(s) that lacks a true nucleus.

Clinical Governance A framework through which NHS organisations are accountable for continuously improving the quality of their services and safeguarding high standards of care by creating an environment in which excellence in clinical care will flourish.

Clostridium difficile A bacterium which can cause severe diarrhoea or enterocolitis. This most commonly occurs following a course of antibiotics which has disturbed the normal bacterial flora of the gut.

Commission for Health Improvement	An executive Non Departmental Public Body, established under the Health Act 1999, which came into being on 1st November 1999. The commission is a key element of the Department's plans to drive up quality in the NHS. Their functions are to: develop clinical governance; conduct a rolling programme of local reviews on the implementation and adequacy of clinical governance; and help the NHS identify and tackle serious or persistent clinical problems.
Community	Related to populations, or services outside the hospital.
Compliance	The degree to which patients follow the instructions for taking a course of treatment or healthcare workers follow an infection control policy.
Consultant(s) in Communicable Disease Control (CCDC)	A doctor, appointed by each Health Authority, who has responsibility for the surveillance, prevention and control of infections within a defined geographical area.
Denominator	The population considered to be at risk eg. the total number of people admitted to a hospital or receiving a particular anti-microbial agent.
Disinfection	To use a chemical agent, which destroys or removes micro-organisms but not bacterial spores. Used to cleanse surgical instruments and surfaces of equipment or furniture.
Epidemiology	The study of the occurrence, cause, control and prevention of disease in populations, as opposed to individuals.
Epidemiologist(s)	An investigator who studies the occurrence of disease or other health related conditions or events in defined populations.

Fungus	A simple plant which lacks the green pigment chlorophyll. Some fungi cause local infections such as thrush and athlete's foot, but may also cause serious illness in immuno-compromised people.
Hospital acquired infection	An infection that was neither present nor incubating at the time of a patient's admission to hospital (the definition used for this study is an infection that normally manifests itself more than three nights after the patient's admission to hospital).
Hospital hygiene	The hospitals routine procedures on cleaning, housekeeping, disinfection, sterilisation of instruments, equipment, production of sterile supplies, safe collection and disposal of clinical waste, kitchen hygiene, control of insects, vermin, etc.
Hospital Infection Control Committee	The main forum for routine consultation between the infection control team and the rest of the NHS Trust. It is required to approve and lend support to the infection control team's programme.
Immune	Being highly resistant to a disease due to the formation of antibodies, the development of immunological competent cells, or both as the result of another mechanism.
Incidence	The number of new events/episodes of a disease that occur in a population in a given time period.
Infection	Invasion and multiplication of harmful micro-organisms in body tissues.

Infection control doctor(s)	Normally a consultant medical microbiologist, with knowledge of aspects of infection control, which should include epidemiology. The infection control doctor normally provides leadership to the infection control team and is responsible to the NHS Trust Chief Executive for its work.
Infection control nurse(s)	Normally a registered general nurse with knowledge of all aspects of infection control.
Infection control team(s)	A team within an NHS Trust which has prime responsibility for, and reports to the Chief Executive on, all aspects of surveillance prevention and control of infection. The members of the team include an infection control doctor and infection control nurse(s).
Infectious	Caused by or capable of being communicated by infection.
Isolation	To remove a patient from the general ward setting to a place away from normal contact with other people.
IT	Information technology such as computers.
Medical microbiologist(s)	A doctor who studies the science of the isolation and identification of micro-organisms that cause diseases in humans and applies this knowledge to treat, control and prevent infections in humans.
Methicillin	A type of antibiotic which used to be used to treat staphylocci infections and is now used in the laboratory as a marker for resistance.
Microbiology	The science of the isolation and identification of micro-organisms. Medical microbiology is concerned with those micro-organisms which cause diseases in human.

Micro-organism	An organism too small to be seen with the naked eye. The term includes bacteria, fungi, protozoa, viruses and some types of algae.
Morbidity	The state of being diseased, or in a reduced state of health.
Mortality	Death.
MRSA (methicillin resistant *Staphylococcus aureus*)	A strain of *Staphylococcus aureus* that is resistant to methicillin and has various patterns of other antibiotic resistance.
Multi resistant	A micro-organism that is resistant to two or more unrelated antimicrobial agents.
National Institute of Clinical Excellence	NICE was set up as a Special Health Authority on 1st April 1999 and as such is part of the NHS. Its role is to provide the NHS with authoritative, robust and reliable guidance on current "best practice". This guidance covers individual health technologies and the clinical management of specific conditions.
Normal flora	The micro-organisms that normally live on the body, also called commensal organisms. When antimicrobial agents are used to treat infectious disease they can affect the normal flora and disrupt their ability to provide protection against infection.
Nosocomial	Hospital acquired.

Outbreak	An incident in which two or more people have the same disease, similar symptoms or excrete the same pathogens, and in which there is a time/place/person association. Also a situation where the observed number of cases unaccountably exceeds the expected number.
Public Health Laboratory Service	A Government funded organisation of public laboratories based in district, general and teaching hospitals in England and Wales, and a central facility at Colindale in North London which houses the headquarters, National Reference Laboratories and Communicable Disease Surveillance Centre. Its purpose is to protect the population from infection.
Prevalence	The total number of cases of a specific disease in existence in a given population at a certain time.
Prevalence rate	The total proportion of cases of a specific disease in existence in a given population at a certain time.
Prophylaxis	Any means taken to prevent disease. For example, vaccination, or giving antibiotics when patients undergo surgery.
Protozoan	A single cell micro-organism that has a true nucleus and a complex and bigger structure than a bacterium. It may be free living or parasitic.
Regional Epidemiologist(s)	A medically qualified consultant specialising in epidemiology and working with a regional unit of the Public Health Laboratory Service Communicable Disease Surveillance Centre.
Screening	Involves taking swabs from patients and staff which are then subject to microbiology testing to determine whether they are colonised or infected by specific micro-organisms eg. MRSA.

Staphylococcus

A group of bacteria which causes a wide variety of infections especially of skin and wounds. More serious infections include bacteraemia and pneumonia as well as heart valve, bone and joint infections.

Sterilisation

The process by which micro-organisms are destroyed or removed.

Surveillance

Systematic collection of data from the population at risk, identification of infections using consistent definitions, analysis of these data and dissemination of the results to those responsible for the care of the patients and to those responsible for implementation of prevention and control measures.

Virus

A very small micro-organism of simple structure, only capable of surviving within a living host cell

Bibliography

1. Report by the Comptroller and Auditor General - HC 230 Session 1999-2000: The Management and Control of Hospital Acquired Infection in Acute NHS Trusts in England. London : The Stationery Office Limited, 2000.

2. National Audit Office Press Notice - The Management and Control of Hospital Acquired Infection in Acute NHS Trusts in England issued 17th February 2000. Available on www.nao.gov.uk.

3. Department of Health (2000). UK Antimicrobial Resistance Strategy and Action Plan. London: Department of Health.

4. Department of Health Press Notice - UK Antimicrobial Resistance Strategy and Action Plan. June 12 2000 Department of Health 2000/043.

5. Department of Health (1999). Modernising Health and Social Services: National Priorities Guidance for 2000-2001 - 2002-2003. London: Department of Health.

6. Department of Health (December 2000). NHS Plan Implementation programme.

7. Forty-second Report by the Committee of Public Accounts Session 1999-2000 - The management and control of hospital acquired infection in Acute NHS Trusts in England. House of Commons: The Stationery Office Limited, 2000.

8. Treasury Minute on the Thirty-eighth to Forty-second Reports from the Committee of Public Accounts Session 1999-2000 - 42nd Report - The management and control of hospital acquired infection.

9. Department of Health: Health Service Circular (2000). HSC 2000/002 - The management and control of hospital acquired infection; Department of Health London.

10. Public Health Laboratory Service News Release - 11 March 1996. National surveillance for hospital acquired infection launched.

11. Department of Health (1999). HSC 1999/123. Governance in the new NHS - Controls Assurance Statements 1999/2000: Risk Management and Organisational Controls. London: Department of Health.

12. Department of Health (November 1999). Controls Assurance Guidelines supplementing HSC 1999/123. London: Department of Health. and Ministerial Press release 1999/0686 - New Framework for managing hospital acquired infection part of a new range of controls assurance standards (22.11/1999.

13. Department of Health/Public Health Laboratory Service (1995). Hospital Infection Control: Guidance on the control of infections in hospitals. HSG(95)10. London: Department of Health.

14. Committee of Public Accounts Press Release by House of Commons 8th November 2000.

15. Plowman R, Graves N, Griffin M, Roberts JA, Swan A, Cookson B, Taylor, L (1999). The socio-economic burden of hospital acquired infection. London: Public Health Laboratory Service.

16. Plowman R.M, Graves N. and Roberts J.A. (1997). Hospital acquired infection - Office of Health Economics.

17. Emmerson AM, Enstone JE, Griffin M, Kelsey MC, Smyth ETM (1996). The second national prevalence survey of infection in hospitals - overview of the results. Journal of Hospital Infection 32:175-190.

18. Alan Glynn, Valerie Ward, Jennifer Wilson, Andrea Charlett, Barry Cooksa, Linda Taylor and Nina Cole (1997). Hospital acquired infection Surveillance Policies and Practice -A report of a study of the control of hospital acquired infection in 19 hospitals in England and Wales, PHLS.

19. Haley. RW, White J W, Ciulver D H, Meade Morgan W, Emori T G, Munn V P, Hooton T M (1985). The efficacy of infection surveillance and central programs in preventing nosocomial infections in US Hospitals (SENIC) American Journal of Epidemiology 121: 182-205.

20. Holtz TM, Wenzel RP. (1992). Postdischarge surveillance for nosocomial wound infection. A brief review and commentary. American Journal of Infection Control 20(4):206-213.

21. House of Lords Select Committee on Science and Technology (1998). Resistance to antibiotics, and other antimicrobial agents. (HL Paper 81-1, 7th Report Session, 1997-98) London Stationery Office.

22. Report by the Comptroller and Auditor General Session HC 254 1999-2000: Inpatient Admissions and Bed Management in NHS Acute Hospitals - The Stationery Office Limited, 2000.

references

23. NHS Estates Guidance - Infection Control in the Built Environment (July 2001).

24. Report by the Comptroller and Auditor General HC 403- Session 2000-2001: Handling Clinical Negligence Claims in England - The Stationery Office Limited, 2001.

25. National Health Service Litigation Authority - Standards for assessing objectives of risk management (2001).

26. Royal College of Pathologists (1999). Medical and Scientific Staffing of NHS Pathology Departments. London: Royal College of Pathologists.

27. Crawshaw SC, Allen P, Roberts JA (2000). Managing the risk of infectious disease: the context of organisational accountability. Health, Risk & Society. 2(2):125-141.

28. Department of Health (2001). Building a Safer NHS for Patients London.

29. Department of Health (2000). An Organisation with a Memory - Report of an Expert Group on learning from adverse events in the NHS. The Stationery Office Limited.

30. Glenister H M, Taylor L J, Cooke E M, Bartlett C L R (1992). A study of surveillance methods for detecting hospital acquired infection. Public Health Laboratory Service.

31. NINSS (2000). Surveillance of hospital acquired bacteraemia in English Hospitals 1997-1999 London, Public Health Laboratory Service.

32. NNISS (2000). Surveillance of surgical site infection in English Hospitals 1997-1999 London, Public Health Laboratory Service.

33. Minister of State for Health, John Denham Announcement that NINSS compulsory- October 2000.

34. Healthcare Acquired Bacteraemia Surveillance: Statement by the Department of Health on the new compulsory reporting scheme (April 2001).

35. Pratt. R.J, Pellow. C, Loveday. H,.P Robinson N. Smith G W and the EPIC Guidelines Development Team (2000). National evidence-based guidelines for preventing hospital-acquired infections: standard principles: Thames Valley University.

36. Millward S, Barnett J, Thomlinson D (1993). A clinical infection control audit programme: evaluation of an audit tool used by infection control nurses to monitor standards and assess effective staff training. Journal of Hospital Infection 24:219-232.

37. National Board for Nursing, Midwifery and Health Visiting for Scotland and Scottish Centre for Infection and Environmental Health (1999). A collaborative report of the findings of a review of current infection control educational opportunities for health care professionals in Scotland.

38. House of Lords Select Committee on Science and Technology Third Report on Antibiotic Resistance Session 2000-2001.

39. Department of Health (1999). Making a Difference: Strengthening the nursing, midwifery and health visiting contribution to health and health care. Department of Health London.

40. United Kingdom Central Council for Nursing, Midwifery and Health Visiting (1999): Fitness for Practice, UKCC London.

41. Handwashing Liaison Group - Hospital Infection Society/Association of Medical Microbiologists/Department of Health/Infection Control Nurses Association/ Royal College of Nursing/Public Health Laboratory Service (1999). Hospital Acquired Infection: Information for Chief Executives - Why you need to be interested! Sent to Chief Executives of NHS Trusts by the Department of Health - March 1999.

42. HSC 1999/049. Resistance to antibiotics and other antimicrobial agents: action for the NHS following the Government's response to the House of Lords Science and Technology Select Committee report "Resistance to antibiotics and other antimicrobial agents". London Department of Health 1999.

43. ICNA and Association of Domestic Management (1999). Standards for Environmental Cleanliness in Hospitals. Tyne and Wear ICNA and ADM.

44. Department of Health Press release May 2000 Alan Milburn MP- Re-issue of Standards in Environmental Cleanliness guidelines by the Department of Health. London.

45. Department of Health (2000). The NHS Plan - A Plan for investment a Plan for Reform: Department of Health London.

46. Department of Health (2000). Hospital Clean Up initiative launched (July 2000).

47. Department of Health (2000). Announcement of autumn inspection visits (October 2000).

48. Department of Health (2000). Results of autumn inspection visits (November 2000).

49. Department of Health (2001). HSC 2001/010: Implementing the NHS Plan: Modern Matrons - strengthening the role of Ward sisters and introducing senior sisters.

50. Results of second series of hygiene inspection visits (April 2001).

51. Standing Medical Advisory Committee Sub-group on Antimicrobial Resistance (1998). The Path of Least Resistance London: Department of Health.

52. Department's response to the House of Lords Select Committee on Science and Technology Report on Antibiotic Resistance (HSC 1999/049) Department of Health.

53. European Union Conference - 'The Microbial Threat': The Copenhagen Recommendations. Danish Ministry of Health and Ministry of Food and Agriculture and Fisheries. September 1998.

54. World Health Organisation (2000). Overcoming antibiotic resistance: World Health Organisation.

Index

index

index

index

137

Printed in the UK for The Stationery Office Limited
Dd 5070327 11/01 74888 Job No. TJ005746